Power and Connection

THE INTERNATIONAL DEVELOPMENT
OF LOCAL AREA COORDINATION

by **Eddie Bartnik and Ralph Broad**

with contributions from Nick Sinclair, Al Etmanski,
Michael Kendrick and international colleagues

Published by the **Centre for Welfare Reform**

Publishing Information

Power and Connection © Eddie Bartnik & Ralph Broad 2021

Figures 1 and 2 © Ralph Broad & Simon Duffy 2012, updated with Eddie Bartnik 2019

Figures 3, 4 and 11 © Ralph Broad & Simon Duffy 2021

Figure 5 © Neil Woodhead & Ralph Broad 2018

Figures 6 and 8 © Community Catalysts CIC 2021

Figures 7 and 20 © Eddie Bartnik & Simon Duffy 2021

Figures 9 and 10 © Derby City Council 2020

Figure 12 © Western Australia Department of Communities 2018

Figure 13 © US Human Services Network, modified by Western Australia Department of Communities 2017

Figure 14 © Ipsos MORI 2020

Figures 15, 16 and 17 © Yishun Health, National Healthcare Group, 2018

Figure 18 © Hywel Trick 2020

Figure 19 © Mark Aldron 2020

Figures 21, 22 and 23 © Western Australia Department of Communities and Social Ventures Australia 2019

Figures 24 and 25 © Western Australia Department of Communities 2021

Front Cover Photo by Kamran Chaudhry on Unsplash

First published August 2021

Power and Connection is published by the Centre for Welfare Reform

160 pp

ISBN print:978-1-912712-38-0

CONTENTS

PREFACE

This book comes at a time of immense change and hardship for very many people through the pandemic of 2020/21, but also at a time of reflection and celebration of the power of people and communities coming together through good times and bad. We are proud to share this new book on the long history, unique design, wide ranging outcomes and long term and future value of Local Area Coordination internationally. A truly person by person, family by family, community by community approach.

The key focus of this publication is the additional learnings since 2015, how these build on the long-term evidence base for Local Area Coordination and demonstrate how it continues to adapt and thrive in a changing world. It is also a celebration of the role Local Area Coordination plays in nurturing individual, family and community strengths and mutual support and the possibilities these offer for the future in our communities.

Building on the original core Western Australia Local Area Coordination foundations and Framework, the last five years have seen an exciting period of intensive international learning, adaptation and growth. This includes moving towards a 'whole community' approach, ensuring easier access and no barriers to early help, increasing reach across the whole system and emerging international collaboration, mutual support and shared learning. This learning has also further improved the understanding and embedding of broader elements, or building blocks, of design and implementation. These are critical to effectively 'getting started', building authentic relationships with people, families, communities and service partners and, importantly, consistency of outcomes, influence, scaling up and sustainability.

We (Eddie and Ralph), with the great support of Nick Sinclair (Director of the Local Area Coordination Network in England and Wales), have worked together over the past 18 months to research and write this book and we feel privileged to have some great contributions from international colleagues. These contributions illustrate the very personal, flexible, universal approach of Local Area Coordination alongside people and families, the power of relationships and mutual support within communities and the strategic value, relevance and power of Local Area Coordination in a rapidly changing world.

Eddie and Ralph's Local Area Coordination collaboration started back in 2000, supporting some of the early national developments in Scotland. This grew to an ongoing commitment to develop and grow Local Area Coordination in England and Wales since 2007, contributions to Local Area Coordination learning alongside NDIS partner organisations across Australia, the recent new developments in Singapore and Western Australia and through ongoing international conversations, conferences and workshops.

This collaboration has now grown to be the three of us, with Nick becoming Director of the Local Area Coordination Network in England and Wales in 2019 and us all working together to share learning, ideas, challenge and support. This set the foundation for the new book that both reflects on 33 years of international learning and the ongoing vision and relevance of Local Area Coordination as a universal, personal, local, accessible resource and support for all people in our communities and a core part of a transforming service system.

When we first started talking about writing this new book, we were excited and daunted in equal measure by the task of authentically reflecting on the long history of Local Area Coordination alongside people of all ages, backgrounds, cultures and experiences in different countries, as well as the positive impact alongside the local communities in which they live and the wider service system. Our big question was 'How can you distil the essence of the Local Area Coordination design and approach and the thousands of stories of person and community led change – the 'what, how and why' of Local Area Coordination, into a short book?'

As it would with any Local Area Coordination relationship, it started with the three of us taking time to get to know each other better. We quickly found that, although we have individually been supporting the development and ongoing delivery of Local Area Coordination in very different countries and regions, with different histories, experiences, aspirations, challenges and diverse and unique communities, our stories and experiences had so many similarities. These reinforced the universal themes of citizenship, inclusion, the power of natural relationships and the importance of choice and control. It also showed the sustained and sustainable value of Local Area Coordination alongside people of all ages

8

POWER AND CONNECTION | PREFACE

and backgrounds (not just according to their service label) and intentional partnerships with both the communities in which they live and the important formal and funded services that serve them, to make this a reality: *stronger together*.

What started as a reflection on 33 years international experience of Local Area Coordination, now in seven countries, quickly turned into a series of rich conversations, firstly with each other, and then with people from a wide range of backgrounds, including local people, families and communities, leaders, service partners and Local Area Coordinators. We were privileged in hearing stories and feedback from people in different communities, in different countries with experience of either having a Local Area Coordinator alongside, or contributing to Local Area Coordination, and creating the conditions for sustainable, positive change: *people power*.

From these conversations and stories, this book started to take shape. We agreed that our objectives were to promote an up-to-date perspective of Local Area Coordination based on our continuous learning around quality and sustainability, inspire developmental action that supports the ongoing creativity and relevance of Local Area Coordination and encourage, support and strengthen national and international leadership and other networks within Local Area Coordination.

Each chapter (except Chapter 4 Stories of Change, written by Nick Sinclair) has been written by Eddie and Ralph, reflecting the core foundations, learning, opportunities and application of Local Area Coordination at the individual, family, community and systems levels. We also have contributions from international colleagues illustrating how Local Area Coordination has worked within very different local communities, alongside people from many different backgrounds and in different service systems.

The chapters are organised to highlight the key themes underpinning sustained Local Area Coordination international development.

These themes include clarity of the purpose and international history of Local Area Coordination (Chapter 1), the 'must haves' of the Local Area Coordination Framework and the maturing connection to whole system reform (Chapter 2), the building blocks for ensuring fidelity and embedding sustainability (Chapter 3), stories of change and impact

9

(Chapter 4), the growing evidence base to sustain 'A Leap of Fact' (Chapter 5), new horizons as a whole community approach, in new countries and as a key community and service resource in a time of pandemic (Chapter 6) and the critical importance of leadership development and learning networks (Chapter 7). Finally, we outline the vision, value and 5-year plan for Local Area Coordination in a post COVID-19 world, alongside people and families, embedded in community and in partnership with formal services.

Our sincere thanks to local people, families and communities who have shared their inspiring stories, ideas, connections and knowledge. This book would not have been possible without their support, contribution and leadership.

It has been a huge privilege to work with and learn from our wonderful contributors from Australia, Wales, England, Scotland and Singapore, bringing to life the individual stories of people and community led change supported by Local Area Coordinators and the stories of genuine service and system transformation driven by change leaders.

This book's focus on the past 5 years of international development of Local Area Coordination builds on the pioneering and foundational work of the original Local Area Coordination sites and leadership in Western Australia and the further national and international developments. Each new area in itself is a pioneering effort and we acknowledge the collective and inclusive leadership that has built, refreshed and sustained Local Area Coordination over this entire period.

Thanks also to Simon Duffy and the Centre for Welfare Reform for 10 years of friendship, support, and challenge to ensure everything we do contributes to (and doesn't obstruct) citizenship and self-determination for ALL people in our communities. Simon's role in this book has been as a collaborator, critical friend, reviewer and publisher.

Our sincere thanks also to Jan Willacy, who has been alongside and contributed to so much of the development of Inclusive Neighbourhoods, the Local Area Coordination Network and wider international conversations and partnerships over the past 10 years.

10

We have been incredibly fortunate to have international colleagues like Dr Michael Kendrick from the United States and Al Etmanski from Canada. They have both provided long term support, critique and inspiration which has been immensely valuable to Local Area Coordination development and we thank them for their broad perspective and deep insights.

Ralph Broad and Eddie Bartnik

11

FOREWORD

by Al Etmanski

Local Area Coordination, three simple words that herald a revolution in how we as a society take care of each other. Three simple words that rebalance the relationship between the natural caring of families, networks and neighbourhoods and paid, professional, institutional care. Too much intervention undermines natural caring and increases dependency. Too little and individuals, families and communities are left on their own to deal with economic realities and changing life circumstances that are not their fault and beyond their control.

Like all great ideas Local Area Coordination didn't emerge overnight. As you will read, it's the product of three decades of practical application in multiple jurisdictions around the world. I've witnessed the benefits of Local Area Coordination in action for most of that time during regular visits to Western Australia. I am impressed by its ability to mobilise neighbourhood and community resources along with those of the state to support individuals and families. I believe Local Area Coordination is a critical ingredient in repurposing our social care institutions. And it is ready to spread just as the pandemic has exposed and expanded for all to see: the gaps in our social safety net especially for people with disabilities, seniors, those who experience systemic racism, mental illness and who are poor, homeless or in an abusive relationship.

To get from where we are to where we need to be won't be easy.

Our social welfare institutions are undemocratic. They are designed: to manage; to ignore natural relationships; to eliminate reciprocity; to restrict eligibility; to enable a few to control the many; to provide order, consistency and predictability; to minimise controversy. To maximise compliance. They turn beneficiaries into 'clients' a word whose Latin root means to follow, to obey. Institutions maintain their monolithic structures with utter confidence in their approach to problem solving even though their track record is spotty at best. And despite the best efforts of talented people who work for them.

Their dominance comes with an enormous social and financial mortgage. The record indicates that institutional decision-making undermines citizen action, ignores community solutions, increases dependency, and preserves resources to maintain out-of-date approaches.

By contrast the task of taking care of each other requires immediate feedback, constant adjustment, discernment and flexibility. Most of all it depends upon genuine, give and take communication. Context matters where people are concerned. The task cannot be divided into rigid, predetermined steps and mass produced the way manufacturing must be.

That's what makes Local Area Coordination the right idea at the right time.

It is a 'one size fits one' bridging innovation. Local Area Coordinators specialise in understanding the challenge from the individual and family perspective as well as familiarising themselves with the way the system operates. They are the link between the assets of local communities and formal service provider organisations and their government funders. They shine a light on the natural ingenuity of so-called ordinary people who have the extraordinary ability to invent themselves out of adversity. Local Area Coordinators act as interpreter, broker, coach, buffer, champion, liaison and sometimes negotiator. And, as you will read in the case studies and profiles that dot this remarkable book, they operate on trust.

Government involvement in social care is an expression of democratic will. Sadly, the institutional apparatus that has evolved treats care as a commodity. Originally designed for nineteenth century challenges, no wonder they struggle with twenty-first century ones. And are enormously difficult to turn around. Most attempts at changing their course have led to piecemeal reforms. Not sufficient to address the flawed assumptions in their original design, nor to eliminate systemic discrimination against minority groups. For example, baked into the disability support system are eugenic principles that characterise disabled people as less than human and therefore unworthy of society's scarce resources. During the pandemic, with a few exceptions, this led to triage thinking. Only when everyone else was taken care of did governments turn their attention to the challenges disabled people face.

Local Area Coordination does not absolve government from its role in ensuring its citizens are adequately taken care of. Rather it repurposes that role. It shifts government's responsibility from producing and financing managerial care to supporting the problem-solving ability of individuals, families and communities, and to removing structural barriers to inclusion.

The potential downstream influence of a small, high leverage intervention like Local Area Coordination is immense. And remarkably inexpensive as the Australian Productivity Commission and other evaluation studies document. There is also a democracy dividend as people who were made clients of social care institutions take back their personal agency and become engaged citizens.

The pandemic has revealed that social resilience is a do-it-together not a do-it yourself project. Which is what Local Area Coordination has been demonstrating all along. This book offers those wanting to 'build back better' after the pandemic practical solutions that have stood the test of time. It provides ample evidence to demonstrate that Local Area Coordination is the key to monumental versus incremental reform.

13

1. Introduction

The Local Area Coordination Vision is that 'All people live in welcoming communities that provide friendship, mutual support, equity and opportunities for everyone.'

Power and connection

Local Area Coordination is about people and the communities in which they live. It's about understanding, celebrating and nurturing the strengths, aspirations, valued contribution, choices and rights of all people in our communities and the power, connections and possibilities of the communities in which they live.

At a time internationally when social care, health, housing and community needs are increasing, whilst available resources in many places are scarce or decreasing and pressure on services is growing, change is urgently needed. It is neither right nor sustainable for the service system to continue to manage 'demand' through a process of people having to wait for crisis and harm before receiving support, coupled with deficit based 'needs' assessments, testing eligibility and deciding service access.

Now more than ever, it is time to look at how, together with local people, communities and services, we can build the conditions for people to stay strong, safe, connected and valued as active, contributing citizens and to re-balance our limited resources towards a greater focus on individual, family and community capacity building and mutual support.

Local Area Coordination, when implemented correctly in partnership with people, communities and the service system, nurtures resilience, personal connections and relationship networks and promotes active citizenship. The increases in self-sufficiency and informal community support subsequently reduces demand for and dependency on important formal services. This is key to maintaining the strengths, mutual support and sustainable local solutions developed by local communities during the pandemic and in building a more effective, personal, local, connected and flexible post-pandemic service system.

Six years on from *People, Places, Possibilities* (Broad, 2015), we are now able to review international Local Area Coordination developments and evidence, especially the universal themes that support and drive individual, family and community led change, resilience and mutual support and whole system transformation.

14

The purpose of Local Area Coordination

Right at the start, we wish to make clear our working understanding of the purpose and desired outcomes of Local Area Coordination.

History has shown that the term can be widely used, but in practice may reflect differing understanding, interpretation and implementation of "fidelity", or what is sometimes referred to as 'evidence-based practice'. Where understanding, implementation and delivery are inclusive, strong and consistent, then the evidence is that positive individual, family and community outcomes and service transformation follows. Where it is not, outcomes and transformation diminish accordingly.

The Local Area Coordination Charter

Develop partnerships with individuals and families as they build and pursue their goals and dreams for a good life and with local communities to strengthen their capacity to include all people, including those at risk of exclusion, as valued citizens.

Local Area Coordination is a long-term evidence-based, capacity-building approach for working alongside people of all ages and backgrounds in our communities. It demonstrates strong multi-level outcomes and value for money when implemented with fidelity.

Local Area Coordinators work to increase the capacity and resilience of individuals, families, communities and service systems and to decrease the demand for and reliance on formal services and funding, wherever possible. Key Local Area Coordination outcomes include:

- Living a rich and fulfilling life, supportive natural relationships, citizenship, contribution, and family resilience
- More welcoming, inclusive, supportive and better resourced communities
- Transformed service systems and more effective use of resources, where services have a stronger partnership with and connection to local people and communities and complement and support, rather than replace, informal and community solutions

Evidence clearly shows that to achieve this, it is important that Local Area Coordinators are available to people of all ages and backgrounds (moving from a 'service label' focus to an inclusive 'whole person, whole community' focus), have 'human size' workloads where they can get to know local people well and build trusting relationships, are based in and connected to local communities and implement a series of connected strategies. Together, these create the conditions where outcomes at the individual, family, community and systems levels are more positive, consistent and sustainable.

Local Area Coordinators work to help people find their own, informal and local solutions first and access to rationed formal services and funding is the last strategy on the list, not the first as is often the case with service systems around the world. This theme of fidelity of design, delivery and evidence will be developed and reinforced in many parts of this book and sits as a critical factor in current and future international development and implementation.

15

A brief history

This is a good time to reflect on our journey with Local Area Coordination with over 30 years uninterrupted learning across multiple countries and target groups. For Eddie Bartnik, it started in the West Australian state government with early reform discussions back in 1986 in response to the desperate need to find new ways of supporting people with disabilities, particularly in regional and rural areas, to build a good life without having to leave their families and local communities. Inspiration was taken from a pioneering group of families in British Columbia, the Woodlands family group, who along with Brian Salisbury, were brave pioneers in the early stages of brokerage and returning family members with disabilities from institutions. Crucial initial support in Western Australia came from visionary leaders such as the Chief Executive Officer Haydn Lowe and Chairman the Hon Ray Young, who supported and nurtured new and sometimes disruptive ideas which, based on emerging evidence, created the opportunity for innovation and sustained change. From the original pioneering and foundational West Australian Local Area Coordination site established by Dr Greg Lewis and Peter Dunn in Albany in 1988, a dedicated, inclusive and consistent team grew Local Area Coordination in a careful and strategic way over coming decades. Local Area Coordination is still operating today with full state-wide coverage in Western Australia since 2000 and now across Australia through the subsequent National Disability Insurance Scheme developments in 2019. Western Australia continues to provide the best example of long-term systems reform with data and evaluations spanning a 30-year period.

By focusing on a 'good life in the community,' evidence soon emerged about multiple layers of outcomes where there were benefits, not only for the individual, but also their families, the local community and the wider service system. Importantly, the cycle of evaluation, learning and regeneration continues with evidence and reciprocal learnings from England and Wales inspiring new developments in Western Australia with a broader population than the original target group of people with disabilities (see Chapter 6).

> *"As with many successful innovations in social policy and social support systems, the Local Area Coordination programme emerged from a combination of contextual, political and ideological realities. It was created partly out of dissatisfaction with existing services, partly from the drive and commitment of key champions, including families, and partly from the injection of new ideas such as the service brokerage experience in British Columbia."*

Bartnik and Chalmers (2007) p. 21-22

The origins of Local Area Coordination and its subsequent development need to be understood from the unique Western Australian context which has a landmass ten times the size of the UK but with a population at the time of less than two million. This posed significant challenges for those charged with the responsibility of developing sustainable support arrangements for particular sections of the community.

Local Area Coordination had its origins in regional areas of Western Australia in 1988 with people with intellectual disability. Over the next 13 years the programme was expanded until state-wide coverage was achieved and all people with severe and profound

16

disabilities in Western Australia gained access to the service (see Bartnik and Chalmers (2007) for a detailed chronology).

Importantly, the additional resources required for this expansion came partly from increases in government allocations and also from the redirection of resources from existing programmes. Strong investments were made in governance opportunities and leadership development for people with disabilities and their families. This helped create the vision and impetus for change, as well as the courage and partnerships to try new things within a values-based framework of 'a good life in the community' and increased choice and control.

Bartnik and Chalmers (2007) note that very strong leadership was required to facilitate the transfer of resources into Local Area Coordination from these traditional programmes and strong will was needed to withstand the criticism that came from those affected by this change. Prior to the introduction of Local Area Coordination many people with intellectual disabilities were relocated to hostel or group home accommodation in the capital city or to one of the large coastal towns, a practice that mirrored the displacement of people with disabilities in other societies. One of the key objectives of the Local Area Coordination programme has been to reduce the drift of people with disabilities away from their families and communities.

During its formative period in Western Australia, Local Area Coordination was viewed by many in the existing disability services as an oddity or optional extra on the service landscape. With the passage of time and growing evidence and strong community support, the programme became an essential foundation for the sector and a major force for change and innovation in the overall disability sector. So much so that when the new National Disability Insurance Scheme (NDIS) was created, the Productivity Commission report on the basis of all available evidence, established that core staffing of the National Disability Insurance Agency (NDIA) would be Local Area Coordinators and planners.

Building on this learning in Western Australia and other Australian states, Local Area Coordination has since grown internationally. This started with Scotland in 2000, England and Wales in 2009, smaller projects in Northern Ireland, Republic of Ireland and New Zealand, new developments in Western Australia and also as a key function of national reform of disability services and supports across Australia via the NDIS. Singapore is now the first Asian country to develop Local Area Coordination, as part of their reform of health services in Yishun Health.

With the growing body of evidence emerging from pioneering implementation of Local Area Coordination in England and Wales, Ralph Broad in his 2012 book *From Service Users to Citizens* started to look at the impact and opportunities of moving away from a 'service label, eligibility and service first' system, which was based on the service label of the person. He outlined the move to a new system focusing on people of all ages and backgrounds - the whole person (their aspirations, strengths, connections, contribution) within the context of their family, relationships, contribution and mutual support within the community in which they live. *Whole person, whole family, whole community, whole system.*

This was followed by *People, Places, Possibilities* (Broad, 2015) looking at the ongoing development, stories, early evaluations and outcomes and future possibilities of Local Area Coordination as a key part of a more personal, local, flexible service system. Early evaluations were showing the high value and contribution to emerging regional and national policies and strategies towards individual, family and community capacity building, the value of friends and natural relationships and building capacity, resilience and natural solutions to aspirations and challenges.

17

In England and Wales, the Local Area Coordination Network was initially hosted within Inclusive Neighbourhoods Ltd, before establishing as an independent Community Interest Company (CIC) in 2015. In 2018 the Network moved to Community Catalysts CIC. It acts as a critical network of shared learning, resources, mutual support and research with a focus on both maintaining programme fidelity and ongoing new learning. There is now also an emerging international network of collaboration, leadership development and shared learning (see Chapter 7).

Local Area Coordination has continued to value and focus on learning and ongoing improvement through independent research and evaluation (see Chapter 5). In addition to the multiple studies across Australia since 1988 and several in countries such as Scotland and New Zealand, there have now been 16 independent evaluations across England and Wales in the past 10 years. New studies are also underway in Western Australia, a major new multi-site longitudinal study is due to start in 2021 in England and a proposed new evaluation in Swansea reflecting learning, outcomes and challenges across the first 5 years and recommendations for ongoing improvement and long-term relevance and sustainability.

The studies have been intentionally wide and varied in methodology, but showing consistent outcomes, including improvements in quality of life, reduced isolation, improved choice and control, better health outcomes and strong financial and social benefits, including reduced demand for and dependency on formal, funded services.

In Australia, Local Area Coordination has a long history of influencing service transformation both at state levels (e.g. Western Australia) and nationally, through the National Disability Insurance Scheme. In emerging sites internationally, we are also starting to see early signs of Local Area Coordination influence on the structure, practice (see Chapter 6) and integration of the formal service system.

In all areas, partnerships with government and non-government services continue to strengthen, simplifying the system for both people and services, whilst also creating conditions for sustainable outcomes, self-determination and contribution. Perhaps most importantly, Local Area Coordination has been growing stronger through a period of prolonged austerity in England and Wales and is currently showing significant individual, family, community and service benefits throughout the COVID-19 pandemic.

"This is about making services human, building trust, giving people the space to be themselves to make their contribution in their community. Local Area Coordination demonstrates that we do care about one another, that we want to be together and to pull through together."

Clenton Farquharson MBE

It is now absolutely clear that effectively designed and delivered Local Area Coordination provides a long-term evidence base that moves from the crisis-service model to one that supports sustainable individual, family and community resilience, mutual support and strong value for money.

A brief chronology of the international development of Local Area Coordination follows:

- 1988 - First development in Albany, Western Australia (WA)
- Successive developments in some other Australian states and territories, notably Queensland, New South Wales, Australian Capital Territory and Tasmania
- 2000 - WA State-wide expansion completed and subsequent developmental stages
- 2000 - Key recommendation in national disability strategy 'The Same as You?' in Scotland and commencement in local authorities
- 2008 - Projects in Belfast, Northern Ireland
- 2009 - England and Wales developments commence (broad social care and health focus)
- 2011 - New Zealand as part of 'Enabling Good Lives' reforms
- 2012 - Local Area Coordination Network for England and Wales established
- 2013 - National Disability Insurance Scheme (Australia) from 2013 incl WA NDIS (broad disability, including psychosocial)
- 2016 - Projects in Ireland
- 2019 - WA Department of Communities Local Communities Coordination from 2019 (broad social care and health focus with the term Local Communities Coordination used for the WA state government programme so as to avoid confusion with the national NDIS Local Area Coordination scheme alongside people with disabilities)
- 2020 - Singapore, Yishun Health (broad social care and health focus)

The international Local Area Coordination experience tells us that, despite differences in political context, geographic settings and target groups, human service systems internationally are all challenged by remarkably similar universal trends such as:

19

- Increased focus on self-direction, personalisation and co-production
- Upstream investments in prevention and early intervention
- Place-based approaches and the importance of connection to community and tackling loneliness
- Value for money, sustainability and evidence, more of a lifetime cost approach
- Safeguarding vulnerable people (e.g. Royal Commissions and Inquiries)
- Cultural competence and reducing inequalities

Local Area Coordination ticks all the boxes and is strongly aligned to contemporary human services policy settings and priorities. Whilst 2020 has seen a dramatic change in context internationally with firstly climate change events and then the COVID-19 pandemic, evidence on the ground so far has strongly demonstrated the strengths of the supportive response in those communities where there is Local Area Coordination in place compared to others where they are not yet available (see Chapter 4).

2. Turning the system

It takes much more than just calling something Local Area Coordination to build and maintain the range of positive outcomes alongside individuals, families, communities and across the service system associated with well designed, implemented and led Local Area Coordination. For any human service to succeed, flourish and be enduringly relevant and sustainable, there needs to be clarity and accountability of purpose, design and practice. It needs to be underpinned by the valued contribution and leadership of the people and communities they serve and attention to reflection, learning and ongoing improvement through evaluation.

We will explore the intentional, multi-element role design and practice of Local Area Coordination, plus the key conditions that support the role, outcomes and sustainability through a new framework for fidelity and sustainability (see Chapter 3). These, when fully designed, implemented, maintained and supported by strong, system-wide leadership, create the conditions for positive, consistent and sustainable outcomes at the individual, family, community and whole systems levels. They address the complexities and obstacles inherent within many service systems that increase risks of people falling into crisis, harm, inequality and increasing unmet need, service demand, dependency and cost.

> "The Local Area Coordination approach, combining strategic, individual and community work is a way for people currently beyond the reach of the formal service system to access support and a way of building people's capacity to identify what would better meet their needs. It therefore both develops inclusion and reduces risk."

Scottish Government (2008)

Key design factors underpinning outcomes

Bartnik and Chalmers (2007) describe some key universal themes of practice that they believe "underpin effective supports and services to individuals and families" (p.21) in local communities. These include:

- Get to know people well over time and develop a positive, trusting relationship and work alongside people
- Staff should be well connected to the local community, based locally in places valued by and accessible to local people
- Hold positive values and assumptions about individuals, families and communities and shift focus and resources to strengths and prevention

- See our job as building capacity, with key aims and self-determination and self-sufficiency, rather than just providing a service to fix a problem
- Ask the right question: "What's a good life?" not "What services do people need?"

Increasingly, these universal themes are reflected in national policy and transformation aspirations in different countries, for example:

- National Disability Insurance Scheme across Australia
- Department of Communities Western Australia 'Key Priorities'
- Healthier Together – Empowering Singaporeans to care for ourselves and one another (Ministry of Health Singapore, 2019)
- Care Act 2014 (England), (Department of Health, 2014)
- Public Services Social Values Act. (England) (Cabinet Office, 2012)
- Social Services and Well-Being (Wales) Act 2014. (Welsh Government, 2014)
- NHS Forward View, (England) (NHS England, 2014)
- The Wellbeing of Future Generations Act, 2015 (Wales) (Welsh Government, 2015)

The evidence shows that good design and strong, connected leadership maximises sustainable, person-led change, strengthens communities and acts as a catalyst for wider service change. These 'must haves' include:

- A commitment to understanding 'where we are now and why' - the conditions that obstruct individual, family and community capacity; resilience; mutual support and self-determination and the unintended consequences of the service system
- The Local Area Coordination Framework – the Principles, Vision, Charter and connected role design required for putting Local Area Coordination into practice
- The connected role – a focus on the 'whole person', simplifying the system for people, communities and the system itself
- Strategic thinking - The emerging opportunities and contribution to wider service change and transformation

21

Where we are now and why

In *People, Places, Possibilities* (2015, p. 17), Broad reflected that:

"Over many years, the health and social care system in Britain has become very complex, fragmented and difficult to navigate - for people, families, carers and for professionals. Arguably it has shifted from the role of a 'safety net' - to provide support in extreme or unusual circumstances - to becoming the default system upon which many rely. This can lead to undue dependence on professional services, which in turn becomes an obstacle to inclusion and active citizenship."

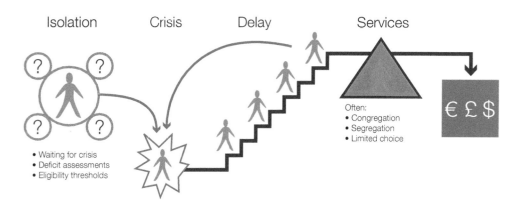

FIGURE 1. **The human and financial cost of a crisis driven system**

The system often waits for people to fall into crisis before responding, assesses people in terms of their deficits (defining people by what they can't do), tests their eligibility for support and then applies services or resources to 'fix' those deficits or problems. For some people in society, the system has 'normalised' inequality, deprivation and waiting for crisis and harm as being acceptable – making the unacceptable acceptable.

This often creates a number of unintended consequences, including:

- Further labelling and stereotyping of people based on their perceived deficits
- Low expectations of individual and family expertise, capability and resilience
- People waiting in negativity, experiencing further harm and increasing dependency
- Time limited, service label specific interventions

These negative consequences often creative a vicious circle: increased rationing of services through increased eligibility (exclusion) criteria, repeated time-limited interventions aiming to 'fix' a problem (rather than build resilience), resulting in increasing dependency, further harm, higher unmet need and higher, increasing inequality and system costs.

Of course, if we only think of fixing a problem or issue for someone, without paying attention to the context of what matters to them, their rights to self-determination (helping people to help themselves), their vision for the future and nurturing their confidence and relationships, they are more likely to repeatedly experience the same issues, but with greater harm happening each time. This is a common theme in many international systems and is neither right, sustainable, nor an effective use of scarce resources.

In the current context of COVID-19, it is evident that there is a pressing and compelling need for change as historical inequities become more magnified. Local Area Coordination is a system and community wide approach that provides an important opportunity to both strengthen people and communities and to start to reduce the increasing pressure on formal services and funding.

22

The Local Area Coordination Framework

The Local Area Coordination Framework outlines the core elements of design, implementation and sustainability that drive outcomes alongside individuals, families, communities and the wider service system. It is underpinned and driven by the **Local Area Coordination Vision, Charter and Ten Principles and connected role statement.** These clarify the wider purpose and expected outcomes of Local Area Coordination, guide everyday practice of Local Area Coordinators to make it happen, support effective and inclusive change leadership and influence wider service practice and change. The Framework is also supported by ensuring the core building blocks of fidelity and sustainability are in place (Chapter 3).

It is based on the proposition that the essence of a good life is the same for any person in society, irrespective of their background or lived experience. This idea creates the opportunity to form the building blocks and assumptions of more personal, local, flexible supports and systems alongside people, seeing each person as unique with strengths, aspirations, hopes and dreams, as well as needs (Bartnik and Chalmers, 2007).

The Local Area Coordination Vision

'All people live in welcoming communities that provide friendship, mutual support, equity and opportunities for everyone'.

The Vision gives clarity of purpose, which then also drives reflection, learning, evaluation (see Chapter 5) and ongoing improvement:

- Are we doing what we set out to do?
- How is this way of working different and benefiting individuals, families and communities?
- Does this include local people as the leaders of change?
- What opportunities does this provide to partners and the wider service system?
- What can we do better?
- How does this influence or support future directions, decisions and policy?

However, it is not enough to just have written values and principles. It requires ongoing attention to strong and principled leadership, values and evidence-based design and effective implementation, ongoing reflective learning, evaluation and improvement.

The uninterrupted Local Area Coordination learning since 1988 has provided a unique opportunity to reflect, understand conditions that enable or obstruct person led change and active citizenship, learn and improve, as well as adapt quickly to be of value in times of crisis or change. The strength and consistency of positive outcomes through Local Area Coordination is built on the intentional combination of these universal principles, key design features (how it is put together and why) and practical ways of working alongside people, communities and service partners to make it a reality on the ground.

23

The Local Area Coordination Charter

The Charter statement describes the purpose of Local Area Coordination to:

'Develop partnerships with individuals and families as they build and pursue their goals and dreams for a good life and with local communities to strengthen their capacity to include all people, including those at risk of exclusion, as valued citizens'

This statement is adapted from the earlier West Australian statement (Bartnik and Chalmers, 2007) to replace 'people with disabilities' with 'all people, including those at risk of exclusion.'

Local Area Coordination is built on a relationship of trust, with the purpose of building confidence, capacity, connections and contribution, rather than seeing people as a collection or deficits and needs, or as recipients of services. When you start with the question of 'a good life' and realise the fundamental importance of valued relationships and making a contribution to each of our own lives and those around us (contribution), it also helps to better understand the limitations, barriers and contributions of formal and funded services.

Curiosity built the map

Rather than asking 'What's wrong with you? or 'What are your needs?', the Local Area Coordinator starts at the start by taking time to get to know each person, understanding their unique situation and personal vision for a good life – 'What's life like now and how would you like it to be?'

It is a chance for a person, and people important to them, to be curious, to explore and plan, to imagine different and better and to take action to make it happen. It creates the conditions for person-led change – person by person, family by family, place by place. It also highlights the critical importance of relationships in each of our lives and things that must be freely given, that money can't buy. This creates significantly more possibilities and is fundamentally different from only being asked a pre-determined set of questions around personal deficits, needs and 'What services do you need or are you eligible for?' It is a key foundation of self-determination, choice and control and citizenship.

Ten Principles

The Local Area Coordination Principles, originally developed in Western Australia alongside local people families and communities, have shaped and driven the design, delivery, practice, reflection, learning, improvement and accountability of Local Area Coordination. Whilst there have been slight changes and variations in language internationally (reflecting local circumstances and culture), the Local Area Coordination Principles retain and build on the original principles from Western Australia and subsequent variations in Scotland, New Zealand, the UK and now Singapore and Isle of Man, where it contributes to the transformation of health and social care services.

The principles reflect universal themes of inclusion and citizenship and are summarised in the table below:

THE PRINCIPLES EXPLORED	WHAT THEY MEAN IN PRACTICE
Citizenship	All people in our communities have the same rights, responsibilities and opportunities to participate in and contribute to the life of the community, respecting and supporting their identity, beliefs, values and practices.
Relationships	Families, friends and personal networks are the foundations of a rich and valued life in the community.
Natural Authority	People and their families are experts in their own lives, have knowledge about themselves and their communities and are best placed to make their own decisions.
Lifelong Learning	All people have a life-long capacity for learning, development and contribution.
Information	Access to accurate, timely and relevant information supports informed decision-making, choice and control.
Choice and Control	Individuals, often with support of their families and personal networks, are best placed to lead in making their own decisions and plan, choose and control supports, services and resources.
Community	Communities are further enriched by the inclusion and participation of all people and these communities are the most important way of building friendship, support and a meaningful life.
Contribution	We value and encourage the strengths, knowledge, skills and contribution that all individuals, families and communities bring.
Working Together	Effective partnerships with individuals and families, communities and services are vital in strengthening the rights and opportunities for people and their families to achieve their vision for a good life, inclusion and contribution.
Complementary Nature of Services	Services should support and complement the role of individuals, families and communities in supporting people to achieve their aspirations for a good life

TABLE 1. The 10 Local Area Coordination Principles

These have greatest strength when utilised in combination. It is not a 'pick and mix', or a matter of using some when we want to and ignoring others when it feels too difficult or time consuming. They guide the design of Local Area Coordination, the role of the Local Area Coordinator, our behaviour alongside people, our practice and how we understand and measure individual, family, community and systems outcomes.

25

Together, these principles create the conditions or building blocks for self-determination, active and valued citizenship, along with opportunities for building and pursuing aspirations. They also highlight, guide and support the range of individual, family, community and service outcomes we expect to see through Local Area Coordination:

"There are core principles that run through Local Area Coordination and define it. If you don't stay true to them, then what you produce will not be authentic and will not produce the same outcomes as Local Area Coordination."

Les Billingham, Assistant Director Adult Social Care and Community Development, Thurrock Council

The connected role – starting from the start

The Local Area Coordination role design and practice is a direct response to the commitment to citizenship for all people in communities, the power of relationships and community, the importance of nurturing the inherent skills, strengths and contribution all people have, as well as the increasing awareness of the unintended consequences of system complexity, barriers and processes that wait for crisis and harm before help is available and then focus on deficits to test eligibility or worthiness for support.

To simplify the system for local people, communities and professionals within the system itself, Local Area Coordination combines a range of connected roles that are usually delivered separately. It has no exclusion or eligibility criteria that stop early help and capacity building, is available to people of all ages and all backgrounds and can remain alongside the person through life transitions and through different parts of the service system and pathway. Local Area Coordinators are located in a number of accessible locations (usually chosen with local people) and mobile within their local communities - a whole person, whole family, whole community, whole system approach.

26

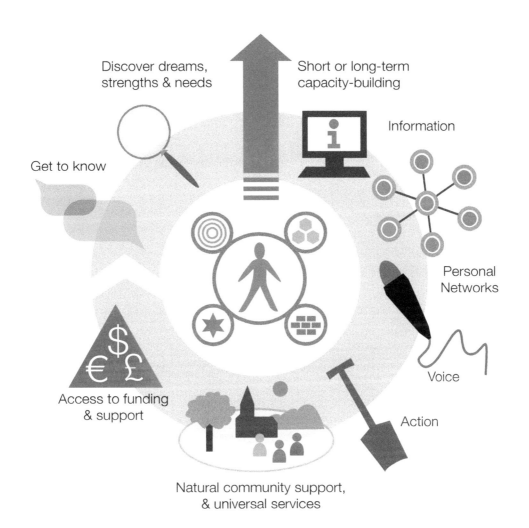

FIGURE 2. **The connected role**

The role combines aspects of access to timely and relevant information, supporting the development of relationship networks, personal self-advocacy, family support, community building, community connecting and support to access, navigate, choose and control supports and services. An accessible 'one stop shop'.

It all starts by building a trusting relationship, taking time to listen, getting to know and finding out what's important – good, purposeful conversations: **purposefully unprescribed**.

1. Explore and discover their dreams and aspirations now and in the future
2. Understand, respect and acknowledge their journey, gifts, skills, experiences and needs
3. Be available to anyone in the community for information, connections or short-term support
4. Be available for longer term support alongside people in that community who may be facing more complex and enduring life issues,
5. Access accurate, relevant and timely information
6. Support people to build and maintain valued, mutually supportive relationships – family, friends, shared interests, shared experience
7. Help people to be heard and have a voice

A REPORT FROM THE CENTRE FOR WELFARE REFORM

8. Assist people to take practical action to do what they want or need to do in life
9. Nurture more welcoming, inclusive, supportive and better resourced communities. Be part of, and actively contribute to, community life
10. Help people to access, navigate, choose and control services and resources they may need

"When asked what difference it had made, Christina said that "no one was listening" to her and "she didn't know where to turn to" for help. It was like I could only get help if things were really bad. Having a (Local Area Coordinator) there made such a difference. She really helped me stay on track and I'm much happier now."

Private communication from an individual

Seeing people only through the lens of their deficits, service needs and service label, risks further labelling, negative assumptions, low expectation, reduced opportunities, dependency and harm.

There is no pre-determined, 'one size fits all' set of needs-based questions, no organisational agenda, or 'prescription' from the Local Area Coordinator. The Local Area Coordinator doesn't have a planned agenda or timescale to fix a problem for the person, or just 'signpost' to an alternative service, nor do they start a relationship by just thinking about an exit plan. Starting with a quick fix and an exit plan, rather than taking time to get to know a person and focusing on building capacity, connections and self-determination, merely increases the risk of higher service use and dependency in the future.

"Compared to other services, the unrestricted nature of LAC support (time and type of person introduced) was considered one of the most important strengths of the programme. Subsequently, LACs affected a wide range of impacts (report section 2.3)."

MEL Research (2016) Leicestershire, England

Instead, Local Area Coordinators take time to listen, build a relationship of trust, explore what's important to the person, acknowledge and celebrate their strengths and experiences, understand who is important to them, understand the challenges they may face and are alongside as they start to build their personal vision and action for the future. These are the foundations of building resilience and supporting sustainable, person led change. By taking a bit more time to get to know and build a trusting relationship, imagining possibilities and exploring the wide range of ways of making it happen, outcomes are quicker, better and more sustainable. One size fits one.

"I felt very comfortable with (Local Area Coordinator) straight away. She really listened to me and I didn't feel embarrassed…she didn't make me feel stupid."

Private communication from an individual

28

STATEMENTS	
Build the right relationship	◆ Trust ◆ Recognising the expertise and authority of the person ◆ A voluntary relationship
Have the right conversation	◆ Taking time to listen ◆ Understand what matters ◆ Understand aspirations, strengths and needs ◆ Understand who is important to them ◆ Imagining better, imagining different ◆ Plans and actions to make it happen
Just the right support	◆ The right type and amount support ◆ Not too much ◆ Not too little ◆ Just enough support for the person to succeed and build capacity, confidence, connections
The right challenge	◆ Supporting people to continue to build their own capacity 'helping people to help themselves', respecting the natural authority, expertise and rights of the person

TABLE 2. **The power of purposeful conversations**

"The Local Area Coordinator never badgered me. If they'd have pushed me, I would never have got involved with the group of friends I have now and I have no doubt that I would still be drinking."

A Derby resident

The Local Area Coordinator role is intentionally flexible, to ensure it remains relevant to the changing aspirations, needs, skills and situations of individuals and families.

"My Local Area Coordinator gave me hope during my most challenging times. I felt suicidal before [they] came into my life and helped me navigate many challenges. Thanks to [them] I am now independent, confident and have connections to my local community. [They are] 'my angel'."

Private communication from an individual

The purpose, reach, practice and flexible nature of the role often poses the question of *'How will we find people with such a broad set of skills and experiences to work alongside people of such diverse age, backgrounds and situations?'*. Local Area Coordinators typically come from a wide range of backgrounds and professions, including: social work, health, housing, education, youth work, nursing, community work, therapy, police, fire service.

When combined as part of a team, there is a rich range of skills, knowledge, experience and shared learning.

> *"A Child Protection Leader noted "once the violence stopped, the work that Local Area Coordinators are doing is building her up to be fully functional, to get her self-esteem back. This particular woman has not come back through our door, no more child protection issues and I think that is directly related to her increasing functioning through working with the Coordinator and her own internal resources as well."*

Western Australia Department of Communities

Local Area Coordinators are also selected in partnership with people from the local community (reflecting the diversity of people within that community). This recognises and welcomes the expertise of, and builds strong relationships with and between, local people, raises awareness of the purpose of Local Area Coordination and embeds an ongoing sense of community ownership and commitment.

By taking time to know people well, understanding their situation, aspirations, interests, strengths, connections and needs, having knowledge of and connection with local communities and a genuine partnership with local people to recruit their Local Area Coordinator, it creates conditions for person led change and multiple positive outcomes at the individual, family, community and systems levels.

Embedded in the community, embedded in the system

30

> *"Local Area Coordinators work in communities as well as with individuals."*

Scottish Government (2008) p.29

Local Area Coordination supports people of all ages and backgrounds to build capacity, resilience and contribution and to find natural, sustainable solutions to aspirations, needs or challenges, wherever possible. However, a Local Area Coordinator can also be alongside a person to support individual and family self-direction of supports, services and resources, where these may be required.

It is therefore vitally important, and of huge value, that Local Area Coordinators take time to build and maintain strong knowledge of, and connections with, both the local community and the range of formal and funded supports and services the people may use or need. This creates the conditions for a shared understanding of what we all have to offer, the limitations and boundaries we all have and to develop and maintain effective working relationships and better, more sustainable outcomes.

> *"Support to individuals who were also accessing formal services would mean that the formal services were better able to focus on their core business as the Coordinator was addressing the underlying and/or peripheral impacting issues preventing people from 'moving on'."*

Western Australia Department of Communities

The power of being 'in and of' community

It is sometimes asked whether the 'community' part of the role can be removed and delivered separately by another person or service. Communities are rich sources of friendship, support and contribution and provide a huge range of possibilities for people to explore. Therefore, having a relationship of trust alongside the person, plus strong knowledge of, connection with and contribution to local community is central to Local Area Coordination and provides a unique, accessible resource for local people. The alternative would be that the system adds in new roles to fill the gap and therefore adds complexity and disconnection back into the system and the experience of the person. Our intentional connections and partnerships with local people, groups, organisations, businesses and services gives the opportunity to build and share our collective knowledge of people, places, resources and opportunities.

You can't be of value to people and families who are disconnected from community if you are also disconnected from community.

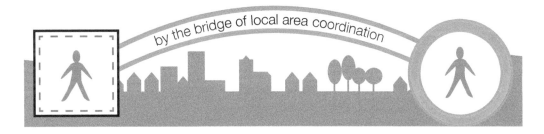

FIGURE 3. **A bridge to community**

The long-term learning has shown that disconnection from community dramatically affects the balance of the role, the relationship with the person, the range of possibilities and opportunities and development of sustainable local solutions, contribution and resilience. It increases the likelihood of returning to a reliance on formal or funded services, the exact opposite of what Local Area Coordination sets out to achieve.

Evidence indicates that a Local Area Coordinator working within a community of up to 10,000 people appears optimum and is most cost effective and value adding. It is big enough to nurture, support, grow and utilise the natural opportunities, connections, mutual support and resources within communities. However, it is also small enough for the Local Area Coordinator to get to know and build effective partnerships with local people, groups, associations, resources, organisations and services. We have found this size population enables more 'human-sized' numbers of people for the Local Area Coordinator to work alongside. If the population is too great, it becomes impossible to build awareness of and connections with the rich resources, connections and possibilities within the community and the level of demand from a bigger area will also disrupt the connected role, thereby increasing the risks of returning to a role that is crisis and service driven.

31

On this issue, Broad (2012) reflected that "Too often services do not just undermine the individual's autonomy, they also fail to recognise the wealth of possibilities that exist in local communities. Local Area Coordination is not just embedded in the community, it is one way of also building stronger community" (p. 17).

"As people concerned with community development they should have a local base where they are accessible to the wider community."

Scottish Government (2008) p.30

"In Western Australia, they have helped people connect with community and thereby minimise presentations at GPs and emergency departments and make connections with other people in their community and reduce social isolation, thereby improving mental and physical health."

Western Australia Department of Communities

When combining the connected role with being locally based in a range of accessible locations (usually identified and chosen in partnership with local people) within communities of up to 10,000 people and having intentional connections with formal and community services, we have the foundations of a highly personal, local approach to building individual, family and community resilience.

"A person called our hub today. No food, struggling with their thoughts and worried about what they would do next. Immediate contact with a MH first aider and an LAC. 6 hours later, they have food, connection to neighbours, support info and a plan to go forward with.

Today's conversation focused on – strengths, assets, new connections, networks and resilience. The person was supported to access information and make sense of that information to fit their unique circumstances both today and for the days ahead."

Neil Woodhead, Derby City Council Twitter message (2020)

32

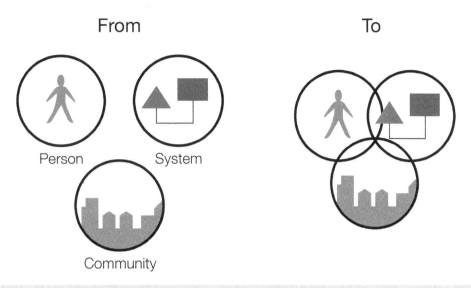

FIGURE 4. **Alongside the person, connecting to community and system**

The wide scope of the role and the deep connections and respectful relationships alongside people, families and communities creates unique conditions for trust and sustainable, person, family and community led change. Where connection with, and contribution to, community is absent from the Local Area Coordination role, or communities are too large, we see an increasing reliance on formal or funded services.

"You couldn't capture much of this in an instruction manual. Local Area Coordination is compassionate, patient, thoughtful and relies on initiative, imagination and great relationship building."

David Robinson, Founder of the Relationships Project

33

Reach across, and partnerships with, the whole system

"They are working with people to resolve issues related to housing and homelessness, ill-health, poverty, engagement in education, daily living, social isolation and more."

Western Australia Department of Communities

For many people, the service system can often feel complex, difficult to access and difficult to navigate. It may require repeatedly having to build trusting relationships with new professionals across multiple services, when moving between services or when going through life transitions. These can often be at times of stress and upheaval.

To make things simpler for people and families (and services), Local Area Coordinators are increasingly available to people of all ages, experiences and backgrounds living in the local community (for example, new sites in Western Australia and Singapore) and they are able to be alongside them throughout their journey, including when receiving formal supports and services, and through life and service transitions.

In *People, Places and Possibilities*, Broad (2015) reflected that "For some people, the Local Area Coordinator may be alongside them through all these times – providing continuity across transitions, helping to build a vision and stay strong; but also there when life gets hard and services are involved" (p. 23). This creates a platform of consistency, trust and support at a time of changing circumstances, changing people and unpredictability.

It starts as the new 'front end' of the community and service support system, an accessible resource embedded in the community with a focus on helping people stay strong and connected as valued citizens, reducing their need for services. Local Area Coordinators work in partnership with local people to mobilise community action and mutual support, community leadership, self-direction and decision making. They can also remain alongside people and families as they use different levels or types of services, at different times of their lives, in combination with and complementary to informal and community supports.

> "A key factor of success is the strong, reciprocal collaborations with local colleagues and services that make the "right" responses available to, and deliver the best outcomes for, individuals."

Western Australia Department of Communities

34

Local Area Cordination supports...

1. **People not yet known to services** to build resilience, reduce need and strengthen community (family, kin & culture) and so **prevent** the need for services.

2. **People at risk of being dependent** on services to remain strong and so **delay** the need for more expensive service responses.

3. **People already using services** to become less dependent, more connected and resilient in their own community and so **reduce** the need for services.

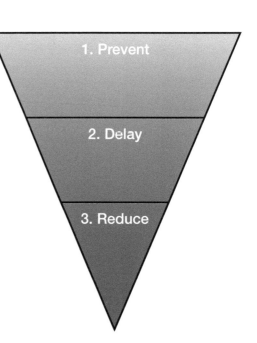

FIGURE 5. Preventing, delaying, reducing – reach across whole system and pathway (the Local Area Coordinator - a trusted person alongside individuals and families as they access, navigate, choose and control services, or through life transitions).

"They contribute to a whole system approach and can help people to access low cost and no cost (supports and) services."

Scottish Government (2008) p.30

This also brings into sharp focus the importance and value adding of effective, purposeful, relationships and partnerships with and between individuals, Local Area Coordination, government and non-government services. This supports quicker, better and more sustainable outcomes, choice and control and individual, family resilience through intentional and purposeful joint working than working separately.

When everything else is changing, the Local Area Coordinator can be a point of continuity, a trusted, ongoing relationship through times of change.

"This was a case that was just spiralling around social work for about 2 years with people not knowing what to do with him… The social work team and the Local Area Coordinator worked together to help this man stop drinking and he is no longer known as a high-risk safeguarding case."

Thurrock Council (England)

Reflections on developing, delivering and growing Local Area Coordination outcomes and sustainability in Swansea (Wales) written by Serena Jones, Executive Director of Operations, Coastal Housing, Swansea:

This pandemic has brought into sharp focus what matters to all of us and going back to the way things were before simply is not an option. Local Area Coordination presents an opportunity to turn the world of community development the right way round.

It is tried and tested, has an international evidence basis and is a genuinely preventative approach – living and breathing the motto 'get a life, not a service'.

At Coastal Housing, we've invested many years in continually studying how systems of work are designed to meet what matters to the communities we serve. And it's the design of Local Area Coordination that makes it so special.

- Coordinators are recruited by citizens in the communities they then work in – relationships are formed from day one (well, before day one!)
- Coordinators are locality, not needs orientated – they relate to people and communities, not problems or labels
- Coordinators are organised around populations with boundaries designed by communities, not authorities
- Coordinators walk alongside people to surface strengths and connect people to others who share similar passions
- There are no thresholds or eligibility criteria
- Relationships aren't time bound or limited
- There is a deliberate reframing of institutional language (introductions, not referrals) – subtle reform agenda is so powerful

35

For the last five years or so here in Swansea, we have worked as a leadership group to keep true to these principles, keep citizens stories and experiences front and centre and have grown local area coordination which meant that when coronavirus hit, the citizen-led hyper-local networks were largely already in place.

The big picture

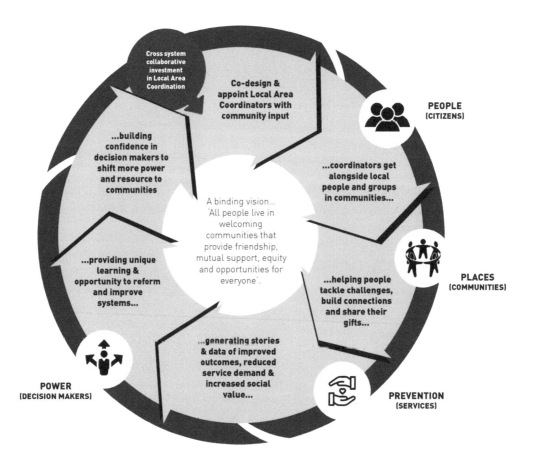

FIGURE 6. The big picture – Local Area Coordination as a catalyst for system wide change. Local Area Coordination Network, England and Wales.

Nick Sinclair from the Local Area Coordination Network has worked with us to develop Figure 6 above to demonstrate the maturing 'big picture' of Local Area Coordination as a catalyst for systems learning and change. Through increased time in place, scaling up and systematic implementation, Local Area Coordination experience and evidence has an increasingly transformative effect in the wider service system beyond those conditions that were needed in the first place to get established.

This virtuous circle of improvement marks a discrete and important step in our learning about the wider impact of Local Area Coordination since the publication of *People, Places, Possibilities* in 2015. It shows the growing commitment of areas to use the person by person, community by community, information and learning provided by Local Area Coordination to drive change across local, state and national service systems.

This involves a stronger emphasis on generating stories and data of improved outcomes, the strengths of personal networks and communities, reduced demand for and dependency on services and increased social value, as well as providing unique learning and opportunities to reform and improve systems. Combined, these work to build confidence in decision makers to shift more power and resources to people and communities.

Some key elements of the virtuous circle are demonstrated through the following sample narrative of questions and outcomes for each of the major perspectives on Local Area Coordination:

People (Citizens)

The question of 'How do I achieve a good, independent life for myself, my family and those I care about?' leading to outcomes where 'We live better, connected lives and know where to go if help is needed.'

Places (Communities)

The question of 'How do we build on the strengths of our local areas and make our places great?' leading to outcomes where 'We have the resources and connections needed to look after each other and our voice is heard.'

37

Prevention (Services)

The question of 'How do we prevent and reduce demand and work alongside people, communities and groups more?' leading to outcomes where 'fewer people are coming to us in crisis. We are working more collaboratively with a strong sense of accountability to local people and communities. We have the capacity to support where most needed.'

Power (Decision-makers)

The question of 'How do we reform our systems and services so they are effective and sustainable?' leading to outcomes where 'Our learning and reforms have taken us to a tipping point for sustainable systems change. Systems have transformed. People and communities adopt more leadership roles, hold more power and resources and increasingly make their own decisions about what happens personally and locally. This, in turn, builds confidence for the overall system to change and evolve'.

Local Area Coordination is built on powerful universal values and principles around citizenship, self-determination, the power of relationships and community, belonging and contribution for all people in our communities.

Its effective design and disciplined practice create the conditions that help to consistently make these a reality alongside people in local communities.

Since first being developed in 1988, the voice of people, families and communities, alongside the many studies and evaluations, has been central in reflecting, learning and improving. It has clearly shown that, where effectively designed and delivered, Local Area Coordination is highly valued by individuals, families and communities (increasingly throughout COVID-19) and delivers highly consistent positive outcomes at individual, family, community and system levels.

These outcomes are determined by the building blocks of Local Area Coordination fidelity of design, effective implementation, scaling and sustainability which are outlined in Chapter 3. The increased emphasis on stories of change, systematic evaluation and collaborative leadership are also highlighted in following chapters.

38

3. Fidelity and sustainability

In this section, we explore some key concepts to support fidelity, sustainability and scaling up innovation. There have been some frameworks from the broad literature that have provided helpful guidance and inspiration at various stages of the Local Area Coordination journey since inception in Albany, Western Australia in 1988.

In the mid 1990s in Western Australia when Local Area Coordination was being expanded over a five-year period to achieve full state-wide coverage, a key challenge was to continue to grow Local Area Coordination into new areas and new times whilst at the same time keeping fidelity to its core features and evidence. Around that time, Collins and Porras (1994) published their book *Built to last: Successful Habits of Visionary Companies* which examined eighteen exceptional and long-lasting companies (nearly 100 years) and compared each one with one of its competitors. An idea that resonated strongly was that highly visionary and successful companies seek to be both highly ideological and highly progressive at the same time. They state:

"The core ideology enables progress by providing a base of continuity around which a visionary company can evolve, experiment and change. By being clear about what is core (and therefore relatively fixed), a company can more easily seek variation and movement in all that is not core. The drive for progress enables the core ideology, for without continual change and forward movement, the company – the carrier of the core – will fall behind in an ever changing world and cease to be strong or perhaps even exist."

Collins and Porras (1994) p. 88

We have found this to be an extremely valuable concept which has enabled a productive tension between maintaining core and stimulating progress to reflect changing times. As stated by Bartnik and Chalmers (2007) "we have found over the life of the Local Area Coordination programme that there is a need approximately every 5 years to systematically review the Local Area Coordination Framework in order to keep it contemporary and responsive to the emerging strategic environment." (p. 34). They also note that this approach was also inspired by the work of Dr Michael Kendrick on safeguarding (1997) who supported Local Area Coordination development in Western Australia during this important expansion time.

39

In addition, it also became clear to us during our various domestic and international efforts to introduce, sustain and scale Local Area Coordination, that in addition to a strong fidelity focus on the internal Local Area Coordination programme itself, a highly strategic approach to risks and opportunities in the external environment is also essential. This is required to ensure that key supports and stakeholder interfaces are maintained and that the programme remains highly relevant and responsive. Mark Moore, in his book *Recognizing Public Value* (2013), sets this out well with his concept of a "public value scorecard for public managers" that comprises three key elements of legitimacy and support, public value (i.e. measurement and evidence) and operational capacity. The upwards and outwards dimensions of 'legitimacy and support' include things like mission alignment with government policy, standing with formal authorisers, key interest groups and media, engagement of citizens as co-producers.

Al Etmanski in his 2015 book *Impact: Six Patterns to Spread Your Social Innovation* provides another helpful lens through which to understand how social innovations in general can be scaled effectively for maximum impact. He argues that three types of innovators are required to achieve long term impact – these are disruptive, bridging and receptive innovators. He goes on to describe passionate amateurs as the original disruptive innovators – "they challenge the prevailing ways of doing things, the allocation of resources, the power and advice of professionals, and the very purpose of a policy, programme or organisation." Bridging innovators are described as "the link between disruptive innovators and the formal organisations and institutions, who excel at spotting the big ideas, then leveraging their connections, reputations and resources to make sure that potential is realised" (p. 40). Receptive innovators are then described as "institutional entrepreneurs or intra-preneurs. Essentially, they are talented and committed bureaucrats" (p. 41). As we read the various case studies of Local Area Coordination, it is helpful to understand how key leaders have collaborated and interacted to initiate, build and sustain Local Area Coordination in each setting through a combination of these three innovator roles.

The 'Building Blocks' approach to fidelity

Bartnik and Chalmers (2007) described key elements of programme quality that were based on the successful state-wide expansion of Local Area Coordination in Western Australia. While those elements have provided a solid foundation for future development nationally and internationally, the context for Local Area Coordination has substantially changed. From a single state-wide government organisation directly providing Local Area Coordination support to people with disabilities through the Disability Services Commission in Western Australia, to a wider combination of delivery mechanisms (i.e.government or local authority provided directly or commissioned externally) and also to a far wider population beyond disability. In addition, there are now several other examples of bringing Local Area Coordination to scale, along with other sustainability learnings where initiatives have either ceased or failed to grow and thrive.

We have consolidated the previous and new evidence base into a new Building Blocks framework that enables a step-by-step building of a sustainable, quality Local Area Coordination programme in each location and jurisdiction. The analogy here is that it is just like building a new house with solid foundations and also the necessary brickwork to keep it solid.

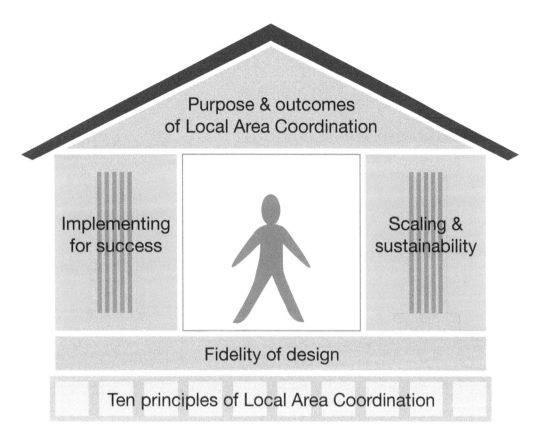

FIGURE 7. **The Building Blocks of Local Area Coordination Fidelity and Sustainability**

Importantly, the first layer foundation of the house comprises the Ten Principles and the roof denotes the strength and security of a network of colleagues and allies. The centre of the house comprises the people and context of each local community which are the key focus of Local Area Coordination work.

Building blocks are grouped into the three major areas of initial design, sustainability and scaling, and effective implementation.

There are nine Initial Design building blocks as follows:

1. A connected role with the right sequence of strategies in a clear job description with high expectations of performance. Not splitting the job up into separate activities.
2. Locally based with presence in, connection with and knowledge of local community - people, places, natural resources. Based in and connected to a geographical community of up to 10,000 (adjust for rural and remote communities). Not supporting local communities from a head office elsewhere.
3. Realistic ratios enable a personal approach to be maintained, with "human size units" so people love their jobs and stay. Ratios generally average 1:40 - 60 for ongoing, longer term support with a range of support needs and ages with adjustment for rural and remote locations.

4. Clear Local Area Coordination values and principles, with the "right relationship" and "introductions" rather than referrals and building capacity not dependency.

5. Credible and skilled external technical support to address all fidelity features, based on the assumption that support needs to be evidence and resource based with a deep understanding of implementation.

6. Whole person and people - not labels, people of all ages and backgrounds, not bound by service label or service specific. Easy access and no barriers to early help.

7. Reach across whole system, simple to access, continuity of support throughout life transition across whole pathway – prevent, delay, reduce.

8. Reach across sectors and ages e.g health, housing, social care, children, adults etc

9. Careful, co-produced selection of Local Area Coordinators involving individuals and families, local people. Move beyond just having a representative on a panel and extend to other key areas of co-production e.g. leadership development, training and evaluation.

There are four building blocks for Scaling and Sustainability as follows:

1. Start small but think big - more than a project on the edge of the system, leveraging Local Area Coordination and evidence to inform system reform.

2. Use of a Public Value framework that addresses legitimacy and support, a public value scorecard as well as operational capacity (See Moore, 2013)

3. Within and cross – sector leadership and creative resourcing involving a combination of recycled and new resources as well as pooled funding from different silos

4. Strengthening of the base of Local Area Coordination, with consolidation of ratios and then building new areas alongside in a connected way

Effective Implementation has the largest number with ten building blocks as follows:

1. Systematic induction and training strategy, strong focus on Local Area Coordination Framework with the connected role and local community connection, preserve core values and adapt

2. Think natural first approach with a greater focus on inclusion and contribution, what people can do for themselves first, how family, friends or community can help, the complementary role of services and funding

3. A personal, flexible human approach, focusing on strengths, local solutions and resilience, rather than deficits, services and dependence, wherever possible

4. A partnership approach with integrated, joint working but always in right relationship with the person, their family and community networks

5. Deliberate investment in leadership, new ideas and partnerships

6. Planned opportunities for regular interaction between Local Area Coordinators and their line managers, 'connected' leadership

7. An open culture characterised by participation, feedback reviews and evaluations, independent monitoring

8. A strong care and rights protection framework and commitment to training

9. Nationally shared values and Framework, regular connections through a Network with international best practice connections

10. Direct provision of Local Area coordination or if external Commissioning then additional safeguards are needed, including options such as public service mutuals.

42

Based on the experience of the past five years, new additions to the original quality framework (Bartnik and Chalmers, 2007) include the requirement for deeply skilled technical support, careful co-produced selection of Local Area Coordinators and within and across sector leadership and creative resourcing. Given the multiple delivery agencies for Local Area Coordination and situations where Local Area Coordination is externally commissioned, there is a requirement for a nationally shared practice Framework and regular connections through an established Network with a focus on best practice.

Each of the fidelity elements and building blocks above are covered in more depth in the case studies that follow immediately below and also as part of the technical support delivered to support Local Area Development through the networks described in Chapter 7. Our combined experience and evidence across all sites and countries is that diluting or removing any of the design features in Chapters 2 and 3 reduces predictability and sustainability of outcomes.

Our Call to Action in Chapter 8 will identify those key strategic directions and actions required to ensure consistency of fidelity, quality and sustainability across all Local Area Coordination sites locally and internationally. This will include turning each building block into an overall self-assessment framework with a toolkit of resources and training.

"We have heard many claim they are already 'doing Local Area Coordination' in one guise or another but this has not been reflected in our findings. Their passion, drive and commitment to the vision and mission of Local Area Coordination is inspirational and it has been a privilege for us as researchers to have an insight into such a powerful mechanism for real change."

Sian Roderick, Deputy Director of Interdisciplinary Research, Swansea University

43

In this section, we profile a mixture of case studies that have been generously offered by key leaders who hold a variety of roles in the broader Local Area Coordination network. Les Billingham and Tania Sitch from Thurrock and Neil Woodhead from Derby City illustrate the consistent organisational leadership over nearly a decade to both scale Local Area Coordination in a sustainable way and also maintain a strong commitment to fidelity. Joe Micheli sets out the careful alignment of Local Area Coordination to the City of York's strategic focus on asset-based areas approach, whereby it is embedded in the broader reforms rather than a tack on project. Councillor Mark Childs from Swansea in Wales describes the important leadership role of elected officials in sourcing integrated funding to fund and grow Local Area Coordination in an environment of scarce resources and competing priorities.

The case studies highlight the fidelity and sustainability building blocks we've outlined and demonstrate the key strategic alliances and alignments needed to scale and sustain Local Area Coordination during times of financial austerity and broader system efforts at reform and transformation. The case studies also reflect a level of depth and maturity where strong efforts have been made over a considerable period to maintain fidelity and grow in a sustainable way, where other sites with the same opportunity may have faltered along the way.

3.1 Fidelity and sustainability in Thurrock Council

by Les Billingham and Tania Sitch

Local Area Coordination in Thurrock was introduced at a time of significant challenge for the public sector. The full impact of Austerity was hitting local authorities. Mainstream services were coming under intense pressure to find efficiencies and there was an expectation that so called non-statutory initiatives would be cut. There was a need to prove the preventative impact of Local Area Coordination quickly to evidence the case for short term investment to secure long term gain.

The last few months of the pandemic have been an even more challenging time for the sector in general and for Local Area Coordination specifically. The emphasis on the shielded population and the need for community-based response has been evident, mainstream services have performed brilliantly but could not, on their own, have dealt with this unprecedented crisis. Local Area Coordination has been at heart of our response, linking in communities and individuals to engender informal assistance and, working alongside social care colleagues to assist with the complex and unique individual challenges that have emerged.

Local Area Coordination locally has been implemented and stress tested thoroughly over the past six years and more recently in the most exacting circumstances possible. It has proved itself resilient to these challenges and able to consistently produce successful outcomes for the individuals supported and for the communities served. We believe this is largely because of two significant aspects of the approach: its fidelity to a set of core principles which provide a spine of consistent and coherent values and the simplicity of the approach that allows for flexibility in operation and adaptability to changing circumstances, two keys to sustainability.

Throughout the initial implementation phase maintaining fidelity to the core principles was challenging for both system leaders and operational staff. In many ways the Local Area Coordination principles were diametrically opposite to a lot of the learned behaviours we, as professionals, had adopted as a result of working in Social Care. The tendency to solve issues for people by following a set of questions (assessment), giving them a service and doing to and not with them had become the norm. 'What are your needs and can you evidence them?' had become the gateway to a service solution, asking people what a good life meant for them was not part of our professional lexicon. We had a 'toolbox of services' that we tended to offer and didn't know the communities in which we worked and what they offered, so never considered them as part of the solution. We, as leaders, found we were constantly challenging others to think differently, only to find we were not doing so ourselves. We also liked to fix things for people. We also waited until they got really bad before we graciously came in and gave a service.

Local Area Coordination has changed that and the evidence in walking alongside people before crisis is overwhelming in every way.

There is something inherently non-hierarchical at the heart of Local Area Coordination, we needed to learn quickly that relationships and collaboration in all things is a crucial part of delivering the core values associated with this way of working. These lessons have served us well in all aspects of our whole system transformation over the last few years. As we moved from what has been described as an ego-system to an eco-system the values at the centre of Local Area Coordination have proved

44

effective throughout everything we have achieved. The difference we see now is that the conversation and language has changed and health, housing and other statutory service professionals and leaders, (who can be the hardest to change as task working and risk averse behaviours are embedded in many aspects of current organisations), are thinking of communities as an asset and challenging their do for, risk averse, and task and deficit orientated starting position. When all people working in the local health and care system and beyond, are supporting communities and individuals in strength based, inclusive ways true change will have taken place.

Maintaining the fidelity of Local Area Coordination remains hard. We are rarely asked to justify the normal services we provide, however, anything transformative remains subject to critical appraisal; now more than ever given the economic pressures that the sector is once again under as a consequence of COVID-19.

The resilience of Local Area Coordination flows from it being predicated upon a strong core set of principles but also on its ability to provide consistent outcomes in a wide variety of circumstances, never more so than over the last few months. The ability of Local Area Coordination to help change the thinking of others is evident, this should guarantee its place as a key part of the future way of providing care and support to people. Finding the strength in those we support is key, but it is also key to find this strength in the system leaders who drive forward change and in those staff who are prepared to embrace new ways of working in extremely difficult circumstances.

We must resist the inevitable pull to move to crisis only responses when resources are challenged and also resist the pressure to dilute or change Local Area Coordination. To assist us all to remain strong and find determination to continue it is important to have a shared vision that all partners sign up to and support with passion and commitment; that has certainly been our experience in Thurrock.

It is our belief that the core values of Local Area Coordination go a long way towards providing such a vision, this explains why the approach has been so successful throughout the world, and why it will be central to us overcoming the challenges we are now facing.

45

3.2 An asset-based approach in the City of York

by Joe Micheli

Power is shifting in York and people are increasingly coming together to define what they want and find new ways to co-design and deliver services collaboratively. People's skills, gifts, talents and networks are being harnessed to provide self-sustaining solutions and a deep reservoir of community resources that people can draw upon to live well. A truly asset-based community development approach to building community and wellbeing. With a thirty-year history of sustained investment in community development, neighbourhood grants for social action and promoting active citizenship, York has strong foundations to build on.

More recently, the Council's Adult Social Care department has moved to a strengths-based approach, recognising its traditional social care services focused too much on deficits and thresholds. Introduced in 2016 a new 'community operating model' has at its core: prevention, early intervention and asset-based community development. This model supports the Council's vision of creating the conditions needed for all people to enjoy healthy, active, independent lives.

The city has deliberately aligned multiple initiatives and models, to enable a force for system change, and a new normal. Shifting away from where social care intervenes at a point of crisis in peoples' lives, often risking dependency, towards a new culture intervening upstream, maximising the individual's agency and their community's capacity to self-manage as the first option, encouraging active citizenship and voice. This is a more enabling, facilitative approach, reflecting collaborative leadership and shared purpose.

York is recognised for being at the forefront of 'Asset Based Area' thinking and continues to invest in evidence-based approaches such as Local Area Coordination. These are increasingly seen as core to system change and not an 'add on'. York's strategic investment in prevention and recognition of the power of community and human connection is opposed to deficit based medical models. The council is finding that Local Area Coordination is providing the foundation for outcomes to be developed. Stories and storytelling have been pivotal to changing culture and behaviours in the system.

Senior leadership within the city at Executive and Senior Management team level has been vital for ensuring the high-fidelity nature of the Local Area Coordination approach has been maintained and the approach grown with communities and citizens across the city. As such Local Area Coordination has proven to be a vital complement to a wider asset-based community development model through building a bridge between excluded people and our thriving communities and making this a reality for all people. That has acted as a catalyst for civic imagination at place level and is proving infectious in the city and service system.

This recognises and respects the power of the citizen and neighbourhood, connecting with people on local challenges, in particular loneliness and isolation. Local Area Coordination has galvanised this action, through adopting a 'person centred approach' helping people build on their own agency and capabilities. Often people have forgotten about their experiences, hidden talents and skills - the Local Area Coordination 'good life' conversation taps into this and unearths passions.

A growing team of Local Area Coordinators now aim to be a resource to all in the places they serve, working 'alongside' people as valued citizens. Community building is a

46

core aspect of the high-fidelity Local Area Coordination approach, helping local people, groups and organisations to develop and sustain their work whilst supporting people to establish new initiatives.

Local Area Coordinators are particularly focused on the assets that exist in communities, building knowledge of hyperlocal, neighbourly, non-service options and potential connections. Where there are gaps, they can support communities to mobilise and establish their own groups and responses too. These 'expert generalists' embody the skills of the 21st century practitioner and specialise in enabling thinking outside the box together with people often on the margins of communities and society. They do not see a 'messy life' rather what can be done and achieved, a 'better life.'

In just 4 years, 3,000 people have been 'introduced' to the York Local Area Coordination team and are now more connected, with new friendships and social networks built, all helping to create more inclusive communities. Stories and language are an integral part of the Local Area Coordination performance framework, helping to reframe the narrative, cultures and behaviours to change and social capital in the city to thrive.

Gavin's story is a fantastic example of an empowered citizen who has overcome life's challenges and is now in control. After being introduced to a Local Area Coordinator, he has become one of York's 70 Community Health Champions, another one of the city's 'impact volunteer programmes'. In his own words:

"A few years ago I was finding things very difficult. I was very inactive, overweight and not washing. There were times where I couldn't get out of bed. Ultimately, I was admitted to hospital with severe depression. Following my release, I started making a slow recovery but medication was not working for me. I came to the realisation that I needed to look at things differently. I came into contact with Jennie, the Local Area Coordinator for my area who I met at a 'pay as you feel' community café, which helped me to connect with others in my local area.

"With time, exercise and positive social interactions, I slowly and surely became mentally and physically strong. I feel fortunate to have my life back and to have turned things around. Because I know how important it's been to exercise, feel good and be healthy again, I want to inspire other people that it can be done.

"In September 2018 I enrolled as a Community Health Champion after Jennie made me aware of the initiative. Following Champion training, I met our GoodGym Run Leader and Move the Masses Founder and have led on new opportunities to support people who are going through difficult times to help improve their health and connect with others. I'm also a volunteer with 'Invisible York' leading tourist walks through the city.

"I look at my turnaround as a minor miracle. Being part of a programme like Community Health Champions allows me to grow as a person whilst having a positive impact on other peoples' lives and I am constantly seeking out other opportunities to get involved!"

The ABCD core characteristics of community mapping, community building and the power of stories are central to the practice of the Local Area Coordination team, who are connecting many other community centred approaches up, and enabling strength based

47

social care to be enhanced. This is a key part of York's journey, community operating model and people helping people ethos. Asset based teams have evolved side by side in York at a time of shared vision and action and informed by ABCD training. This has been deliberate; reflecting the strategic vision within York that ensures collaboration is a golden thread. Importantly it creates a two-way, reciprocal bridge to the Voluntary Community and Social Enterprise (VCSE) and statutory sectors, enabling a flow of new volunteers, sense of good neighbourliness, wider sense of connection and being part of something bigger. A genuine 'asset-based area' and city of service.

We have explored as a council how the 21st century public servant needs to be one informed by values of social justice, equality and trust, and who see facilitation of active citizenship as a first point of action not the design of top-down services. Rather, the council remains committed to the future of public services that are co-produced and 'people powered' with social action as the norm rather than the exception. All informed by the values of ABCD and community building. Local Area Coordination and these examples are just part of this ever-growing movement which is inverting traditional service systems and relocating power to where it belongs, with citizens!

"By using Local Area Coordination as a way to build relations with, and listen to citizens and communities, the council and our health partners have started to understand what is working well and what isn't across our city. We are using this learning to change and improve the systems that are getting in the way of our vision of an asset-based area that starts with people. We describe this as a citizen-led movement of community development, where we will empower people to find solutions that work for them, and where we strive and enable, rather than direct and prescribe."

A Citizen Led Movement - Joe Micheli, City of York Corporate Director for Health, Housing & Adult Social Care

3.3 Integrated funding sources in Swansea

by Councillor Mark Child

Whatever the pros and cons of the argument about investing in prevention, it is easier to get agreement that this is a mutually good thing from friends and partners than it is to get a financial contribution from them. You can see how this could easily lead to assertions that 'This is Council's idea, it is their responsibility, we are having enough problems with our own internal finances without choosing to give the Council money, that would just make things worse.'

There is a disconnect between knowing an action would reduce demand on your scarce resources and improve outcomes for your clients; and spending your organisation's money on it.

In Swansea, within the Council, a few of us were convinced Local Area Coordination was the best way forward. So, we set out to have a Local Area Coordinator for every community and individual in Swansea. Given this belief, we wanted it implemented as soon as possible. There are two ways of funding: core funding or grants and other external sources. If a post is core funded it takes on greater permanence and security, but to divert core funding from a decreasing pot due to austerity, in the face of increasing demand for current services, was going to be a slow and difficult process. Not that we haven't done this, with a level of success, but it didn't answer the "as soon as possible" goal.

The first 3 posts were funded using the Intermediate Care Fund moneys from Welsh Government. This has since changed into the Integrated Care Fund, but we have still used it. This is a 3-year limited pot and wasn't going to get us to our target of 22 Local Area Coordinators.

We knew multiple other organisations had to be looking for prevention initiatives, and would benefit directly from Local Area Coordination, so we decided on a direct approach. To be honest, we expected a respectful and sympathetic hearing and little else.

That is not what happened, all three of the Registered Social Landlords (RSL) in Swansea agreed that Local Area Coordination was great and committed finance to it, enough for an additional Local Area Coordinator. Since then, one RSL has come to the Council with a desire to improve an impoverished area where both have significant housing, in which they committed to increase payment for Local Area Coordinators in Swansea if one could be provided in their area. This added another Local Area Coordinator. I can't tell you how happy we were when we left the first meeting with a commitment, it was before COVID-19, and we hugged.

As a response to the *Future Generations Act* (2015), we gained a commitment from partners that Local Area Coordination was a key element of the shared response. Having done this we then said, 'Well how much are you able to contribute?' Of the two who I think should have said yes, one did, and that meant one more Local Area Coordinator.

As part of an initial evaluation the University of Swansea undertook, they became regular attenders at our Joint Implementation Group. Following their report, glowing, we just said, 'You have loads of students living in Swansea, and many employees, you are embedded in our communities, would you like to contribute?' They said yes, that was another Local Area Coordinator.

This didn't always work, as a direct approach to Health initially failed. But with growing appreciation of Local Area Coordinators from GPs, Community Mental Health Teams,

49

Hospital discharge, community health initiatives, Public Health etc, we have managed to change this to a degree. We have also used the Transformation Fund that is part of *A Healthier Wales*, which is jointly bid for between Health and Local Authorities. We have included Local Area Coordination, and this has come back with initial success and anticipated more in future phases, which means two more Local Area Coordinators now and potentially another three.

Alongside this, the Council has been increasing funding and moving in core funding so now we have a team of 22 Local Area Coordinators in Swansea. This approach has allowed us to increase the numbers far quicker than otherwise, brought many other partners on-board in understanding and supporting Local Area Coordination, which in turn makes Local Area Coordinators' work easier with the communities.

However, this approach hasn't been without difficulties. All Local Area Coordinators start on temporary contracts, often less than 3 years, which may affect recruitment. Occasionally funding dries up without replacement being available, meaning ending a Local Area Coordinator appointment, and withdrawing from an area. This is thankfully rare, but it is most difficult to deal with. Once they are in an area, the good they do is readily apparent, they are valued by all and they have people they are walking alongside. I have had to promise on my life that the next funds I get my hands on will go to replacing the lost Local Area Coordinator. It means you are always looking at ways to obtain funding.

You also come up against brick walls, I have failed to win the argument that Housing Revenue Account monies could legitimately be spend on Local Area Coordinators, police will not (yet) commit despite Police Community Support Officers and others community officers having a very close and symbiotic relationship across Swansea.

One avenue we are planning to explore is that of Corporate Responsibility, the University has been pushing this idea, but we couldn't think of a way in as there were no existing shared structures and relationships. However, through the pandemic, businesses of all sizes have contributed help to local communities, through donations of money, or materials, or employees time, or facilities, and we are collecting all their names, to say thank you and then to see if we can translate this into a longer-term link with their communities via Local Area Coordination.

3.4 Starting small, thinking big in Derby City

by Neil Woodhead

Derby began its Local Area Coordination journey in the summer of 2012 when our first two Local Area Coordinators began the process of getting to know their new communities. This was the culmination of 8-12 months work with Inclusive Neighbourhoods Ltd to prepare the ground for the introduction of Local Area Coordinators into our communities. The time, taken up front to intentionally connect with key people within communities has and continues to pay off, as we now see Local Area Coordination in the city use the 'start small, think big' mantra to carry us to being in a position to able to offer an all-age, city-wide service in 2020.

Whilst this is an incredibly proud moment for us, our journey has not been a smooth one. However, early on in our development Eddie Bartnik talked to strategic leaders about the absolute critical importance of staying true to the key values and principles that underpin our approach, 'Core principles lead to consistent outcomes.' This values-driven approach allied to strong, collaborative design and leadership, connection to community and recruiting the right people alongside residents, has seen Local Area Coordination grow strong roots in our city.

When looking back at the early challenges we faced as a programme, a few key ones remain today, most challenging of all being the ongoing demonstration of the impact this highly relational, connected, community rooted approach can have across the service system. Eight years into our work, there is no doubt of the impact Local Area Coordination can have. Its benefits are felt across all stakeholders; from individuals who are struggling to make sense of their circumstances, isolated families lost in system pathways and processes, communities that have lost connection to their capacity to care through to overly bureaucratic services who are often isolated in the communities they try to serve with ever decreasing financial resources.

The key to this challenge would appear to be one that unlocks several doors. It's all about relationships. With residents, communities, and wider stakeholders. These are relationships that require ongoing dialogue, humility, and a willingness to learn, adapt and respond based on what we hear when we talk to people.

Looking back at the development of the team over the last 8 years, I don't think that there was one specific tipping point that changed the position of Local Area Coordination in the city, more a combination lock that has required the right numbers slotting into place. The most significant being the point at which we as a team changed our mindset from one of constantly trying to prove our case and compete, to becoming more self-assured, generous, and confident in our places and abilities. Certainly, the evidence for 'Why Local Area Coordination?' is now in place and we turn our collective attention onto 'How?'

In Derby, the next few months and years will be an interesting one as we move towards becoming a demonstration site for the Department of Education following the success of our work with young people who have experience of the care system. This, alongside some fixed term work we have been doing with our local Clinical Commissioning Group around people who find themselves reliant of expensive emergency health services, means we are well placed to begin to embed the Local Area Coordination approach across service silos and budget lines based on strong quantitative and qualitative data.

The recent development of information sharing agreements with key partners has been crucial to this.

The constant demand over the last 8 years, to service slightly different funders is a time consuming one that distracts from our core purpose and is the big challenge facing all the programme nationally. The COVID-19 pandemic has also increased the focus on Local Area Coordination as a key partner to get to see first-hand the impact that our service has had, with its strong links and connections to residents and local community networks. This also presents us with a challenge as it is crucial that we avoid breaking the approach by over-stretching the team.

52

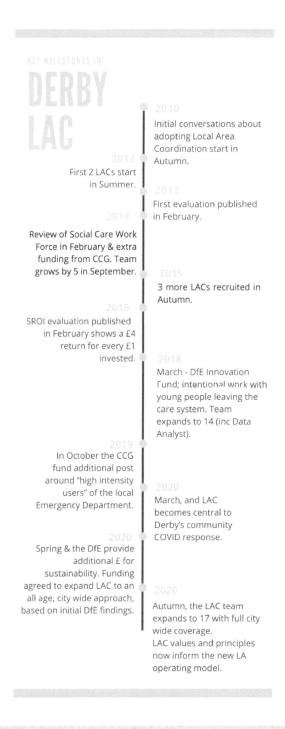

KEY MILESTONES IN

DERBY
LAC

2010
Initial conversations about adopting Local Area Coordination start in Autumn.

2012
First 2 LACs start in Summer.

2013
First evaluation published in February.

2014
Review of Social Care Work Force in February & extra funding from CCG. Team grows by 5 in September.

2015
3 more LACs recruited in Autumn.

2016
SROI evaluation published in February shows a £4 return for every £1 invested.

2018
March - DfE Innovation Fund; intentional work with young people leaving the care system. Team expands to 14 (inc Data Analyst).

2019
In October the CCG fund additional post around "high intensity users" of the local Emergency Department.

2020
March, and LAC becomes central to Derby's community COVID response.

2020
Spring & the DfE provide additional £ for sustainability. Funding agreed to expand LAC to an all age, city wide approach, based on initial DfE findings.

2020
Autumn, the LAC team expands to 17 with full city wide coverage. LAC values and principles now inform the new LA operating model.

FIGURE 8. **Key milestones in Derby Local Area Coordination**

4. Stories of change

In this section we present a mixture of stories that have been generously offered from people Local Area Coordinators have been alongside. It is our intention that these stories will bring to life the theory and discussion that we have outlined in the previous sections and help build an understanding of the difference Local Area Coordination is making. To support this, we have added some summary analysis at the end to highlight the wider narrative.

Stories have a powerful role in Local Area Coordination. It is each person's story and there is value in helping the person to reflect on their own journey and to celebrate the changes they have made in his or her own life. In addition, with permission, the stories and are routinely used for reflective practice and system wide learning. They can also be a vehicle for citizens to speak truth to power and for leaders to bear witness to the impact of systems on people and communities. When shared with intention and to a receptive audience, they can help us to reflect, build a sense of shared accountability and provide opportunity to move with confidence towards a vision of better through collaborative action.

The 7 stories presented here are from Local Area Coordination sites all over the world, written together by the person involved and the Local Area Coordinator and shared with consent. Names have been changed to ensure privacy.

1. Sally shows the power of speaking up, written by Jennie Cox
2. Rishelle gets a brighter start to life, written by Ewa Neal
3. James escapes the 'high intensity user' label, written by Kathryn Humptson
4. Henry and Jess strengthen their relationship, which others said would never work, written by Catherine Viney
5. Michelle works to make her family stronger, written by Mary Flynn
6. Carl goes from 'mental health service user' to citizen, written by Anne Robinson
7. Gemma works to get her child back, written by Kim Harris

Some are from areas who have been leading Local Area Coordination for many years, some much newer. Some are about Local Area Coordination in a more rural context, some more urban. What the stories will highlight is that, where it has been designed properly, the outcomes are remarkably similar, regardless of the age and background of the individual or the context of the community or country in which they live. This consistency of outcomes is not just for people and their families, but also for their communities and the strategic aspirations of the wider service infrastructure surrounding them.

53

Ultimately, these powerful individual stories help to highlight the much bigger overall narrative of Local Area Coordination:

- If Local Area Coordinators are present and take time to get to know the whole person, their family and community, then they can support in a way that truly builds capacity or reduces 'problems' that will be costly to people, their communities and systems
- With the practical, balanced support of Local Area Coordinators alongside them, people start to move towards their vision of a better life, finding the space to make connections, share their gifts and their contribution in society
- This amplifies social value and grows community
- The stories that speak to this happening inspire trust and confidence for people to drive systems reform, increase collaboration and ensure more resource flows directly to people, families and communities
- Ultimately this helps to shape more resilient, collaborative and connected systems that are built on the natural authority of citizens, families and local communities rather than siloed service responses based on an increasingly high eligibility threshold

You will see from the stories we shared here that they speak to the range of key enabling conditions designed in Local Area Coordination, for instance:

- Ease of access
- Range of ways of connecting or being introduced
- Behaviours (making time to listen and understand the big picture)
- Focus on strengths
- Knowledge of connections with contribution to community.

The stories also show multiple beneficiaries – the person, their family and those who are important to them, the community in which they live, work, meet-up and the service system. All will have a different experience of the journey, but the multi-layered outcomes are something that is unique to Local Area Coordination and often not understood in a system that focuses on simple, system driven outputs with a single and siloed purpose.

"Working with my Local Area Coordinator has not only made me want to live, it has for the first time in years, made me start to see there is a future. It has helped me come from feeling that I am completely useless, to realising that I do have qualities and I do deserve a life."

Recent feedback from citizen of Swansea

4.1 Sally shows the power of speaking up

by Jennie Cox

Sally, 29, was introduced to Local Area Coordinator Jennie by her mum and older sister. The family were experiencing complex issues related to a long history of trauma and domestic abuse. Sally was in a difficult place but trusted Jennie as she was recommended by her family.

Sally soon opened up about some of the things going on in her life. Sally was living as homeless – she'd been allocated a flat by the Council, however, she had felt unable to stay there due to anti-social behaviour from her neighbour.

Sally had raised complaints about her neighbour but felt her Housing Officer wasn't listening. The noise from this flat and aggressive response when she had confronted the man making it, had triggered traumatic memories of violence from Sally's childhood which had triggered a mental breakdown. Sally was unable to go to work and was signed off sick. She'd worked at a children's nursery for over nine years and loved her job. Her life was turned upside down and she was suddenly anxious and emotional most of the time. Sally's vision of a good life was for things to go back to normal, to have a safe home and return to a job she loved. Jennie and Sally agreed a plan together through the Local Area Coordination 'Shared Agreement.'

Jennie helped Sally to explain to the Council Housing department that although they saw her as 'adequately housed' it was a lot more complicated than that. They arranged a meeting so Sally could be heard. Her sister also attended, to explain the wider family context. Unfortunately Sally and her sister's frustration was misinterpreted as 'challenging behaviour' and she met a defensive and punitive response initially. Her Housing Officer raised a separate historical issue as possible breach of tenancy. Sally felt he was dishonest and unfair in this exchange, which led to a fundamental breakdown in relationship and a long process to reach a resolution. Jennie walked alongside Sally and her family through this process, making sure their voices were heard at every step and encouraging a reframing of her situation in a compassionate way. After several conversations up to a senior manager level, Sally and Jennie were able to work collaboratively with housing managers to arrange a discretionary move to a new home on the same estate as her mother and sister. This took several months and only when this happened was Sally able to start really rebuilding her life.

Jennie helped Sally with accessing specialist support for her mental health and possible Autism diagnosis. Jennie also helped Sally claim benefits when statutory sick pay ended and liaise with her employer about getting back to work. They attended meetings at the Nursery, where her employer showed little compassion or understanding of mental health issues, questioning whether she was 'fit to work with children at all.' Ultimately Sally was unable to return to work as the relationship with her manager irrevocably broke down. Jennie helped Sally seek advice from the Advisory, Conciliation and Arbitration Service (ACAS) about options and negotiate a Settlement Agreement on the grounds of discrimination under The Equalities Act. Sally received financial compensation, agreement to end employment on mutual terms with a positive reference and a significant amount of owed holiday pay. All of this helped her towards starting afresh when she felt ready, working with children, doing what she loves and is good at.

55

After all of this, Jennie attended a meeting with housing managers to feedback on Sally's experience and explore lessons that could be learned from Sally's story. This has now developed into monthly meetings to share experiences of other people the Local Area Coordination team have been walking alongside and look at positive system change that can be made based on real life stories.

Sally has settled into her new home and is passionate about social justice and housing rights. Her confidence has grown and she recently won an appeal independently, overturning a decision about Personal Independence Payments. She takes opportunities to make things better for other people through telling her story and helping to link others to advice. She has introduced some of these people to other Local Area Coordinators across the city and together they are currently making her story into a short film together with a local mental health charity. Sally now wants to help anyone avoid a situation like the one she found herself in.

Critical outcomes for Sally and the system include:

- Having one consistent and trusted person who could help with all of it was key for Sally to get her life back on track
- The Local Area Coordination rights-based approach focused on Sally's vision of a good life helped her find a voice and challenge discrimination. She now feels heard and empowered to work towards change to help others
- The support from Jennie prevented Sally experiencing a more severe mental health crisis which could have led to hospital admission and possible suicide, something that she had talked about
- Homelessness was prevented for Sally through advocacy to challenge decisions and for others through wider system change to improve the way housing services will be delivered in future. Sally knows her story was a catalyst for these changes and is proud of this.

"Housing Services work with the Local Area Coordinator Team on a growing number of cases, we have achieved some really positive outcomes for people and built solid relationships with the team. We have used case studies and people's stories as a way of learning how we can shape our services in a more person centred way and when we are reviewing policies and developing new initiatives."

Rachael Bassett – City of York Council Housing Services Change Manager

4.2 Rishelle gets a brighter start to life

by Ewa Neal

Rishelle was introduced to Kerry (Local Communities Coordinator) through the Department of Housing Team Leader after accepting an offer of a public housing unit. The Housing Team Leader highlighted some concerns, particularly her young age of 17 years. Kerry was advised Rishelle had been homeless from 15 years of age, was engaged with short term accommodation options last year, identified as Aboriginal, on a Youth allowance, was studying in year 11 at a local College and connected to GP Outreach services for anxiety and depression (but not utilising the service). Because she had no belongings of her own, Housing Services had arranged some financial assistance, furniture and household items through various Outreach services.

Rishelle initially shared bits of her life with Kerry however as she became more trusting over time shared a lot more, giving Kerry the depth and understanding of what was truly important to her. Rishelle's story is a very complex one. There has been a lot of grief, trauma, substance abuse, poor mental health, involvement of child protection service and contact with the justice system. In 2016, her father suddenly passed of cancer. In 2018, her 10-week-old niece passed of Sudden Infant Death. In December 2019, her mother was released from prison where she was serving a sentence for drug offences. Rishelle disclosed to Kerry that she smokes marijuana to assist her with sleeping and she has had to call the police when her 'on and off' partner damaged property in the home. Rishelle was struggling to pay her rent, had unpaid fines, overdue utilities bills and was finding it difficult to attend school.

Rishelle was wanting support to help her get on top of these issues, to be able to get her driver's licence and finish school. It was found that Rishelle was on the wrong welfare benefit which was requiring her to report to an employment agency even though she was a full-time student. Rishelle really wanted to graduate from school and break the cycle by getting a qualification in hairdressing. She also wanted to reconnect with the Doctor's Outreach service to support her with her mental health.

For various reasons the initial connection with Kerry was difficult at times. Kerry persisted with letting Rishelle know she is there as needed, by phone and visits, to reiterate the support was voluntary and ask whether she wanted to continue with her input. Rishelle was very grateful for the concern and over time, and as trust developed, started connecting with Kerry.

Kerry supported Rishelle to identify issues, plan what was needed and who she needed to connect with to address them. She also supported Rishelle with information and connecting her with the right supports and services for her. Over time, Kerry helped Rishelle gain a good understanding of her rights and responsibilities as a tenant and helped her to develop connection with the local Housing office and confidence in dealing with the housing officers.

Rishelle is now able to address any issues with her housing officer directly, and only lets the Kerry know what she has achieved, instead of needing her presence at the meetings.

Kerry also supported Rishelle in connecting with Centrelink to change her payments so she is receiving the correct financial assistance, allowing her to attend school. Rishelle is now planning for school engagement for the new year having a planned meeting with the

57

College at beginning of the school year 2020 to ensure she knows what she needs to do in order to complete the year.

Kerry has also supported with accessing food parcels to make sure when her mother and other relatives visit over the Christmas and New Year period she had enough food.

Kerry continues to be involved in Rishelle's life, through its ups and downs, supporting her in accessing information and supports and reassessing her goals and needs.

Recently Rishelle has identified she is ready to address her mental health and drug and alcohol use. Local Communities Coordination supported her in connecting with the right services and Rishelle is following through.

Rishelle's personal relationships are very complex and currently her connection with her family members has broken down. Kerry was able to support Rishelle with informal connection to another woman, a strong local person in her early 30s, well connected and active in her local community, who has past lived experience similar to Rishelle's, is also aboriginal and can be a strong role model. Rishelle is a very private person and does not connect with others easily, but she has decided to connect with the woman, who can be there in times of crisis, as well as in times of celebrations. Rishelle and the woman are currently planning to connect Rishelle to a group of aboriginal women with similar interests.

Rishelle now has an understanding of the responsibilities of having to manage her financial commitments in order to prevent her losing her home and a bad credit rating. Rishelle can manage her tenancy directly with housing officers as needed and has peace of mind that she is keeping up to date with her payments. It has also raised an awareness for Rishelle at looking at casual work to supplement the pension as she is aware that her options "to go places and buy stuff" are limited due to having little money.

The support from Kerry, at a stage when escalation was likely, has avoided an eviction and potential homelessness and is helping improve Rishelle's credit rating. Through Kerry's support, Rishelle is connected to some natural supports which are helping to avert her reliance on formal services, support her wellbeing, and strengthen her circle of people who care about her, can help in difficult times and share in joy of shared interests and celebrating success. Rishelle is also now seeking the assistance she needs for her mental wellbeing. She is better able to take control of her situation and maintain her independence.

Rishelle wishes for Kerry to remain that constant person in her life to assist and support her going forward together.

Critical outcomes for Rishelle include assistance to:

- Build, strengthen and turn her life around
- Increase her school attendance and supporting her educational achievements towards a hopeful future of career and employment
- Avoid eviction and homelessness
- Self-manage her tenancy and finances and build an effective relationship with Housing services
- Increase her confidence, capacity, choice and control over decisions, supports and services
- Build natural, supportive relationships in her community
- Connect with women who have shared interests
- Reduce her court appearances for housing tenancy issues and unpaid fines
- Reduce Police call outs through having financial issues minimised, increased awareness of bad and good relationships thus leading to better relationships

- Access relevant information and food
- Reduce her need for Local Communities Coordinator support, but she knows it is easy to access in the future

Some key outcomes for services include:

- Reduced need for formal services through building natural, relational supports in her community
- Reduced admissions to mental health through been assisted and supported by LCC by addressing other areas of her life to minimise stress and anxiety
- Avoided eviction
- Rishelle is receiving the correct pension therefore reducing the need for other benefits

The example also delivers on key government priorities around Aboriginal well-being: *A Bright Start for Children and Housing.*

"Housing Support Officers can do the tenancy part - but their workloads don't allow them to be able to put the time in to sort out other issues. The gold part about the LCC is being able to put in the time to stop people from getting lonely and isolated."

Western Australia Department of Communities

59

4.3 James escapes the 'high intensity user' label

by Kathryn Humptson

James was introduced to Local Area Coordination by his Local Housing Officer. He was struggling to maintain his tenancy, manage his property and budget his money. He had also fallen out with most of his neighbours over the state of his garden. At the time of introduction, he was in the process of being evicted and was refusing to engage with services and other people.

James has no family. Prior to introduction, he was addicted to alcohol. His drinking and loneliness often caused him to neglect himself; he would go days without food. On one occasion, James was found collapsed in the street. A passer-by called an ambulance and he was admitted to hospital.

James was not managing his long-term health conditions. As a result of his drinking and his self-neglect, he was making frequent calls for an ambulance which often led to hospital admissions. There were safeguarding concerns for James because of these problems. His vulnerability also caused him to be at risk of abuse. As a result of these problems, the police were sometimes called-out to see James.

Over a period of months, James and his Local Area Coordinator, Emily, developed a good, trusting relationship. He allowed Emily into his home and they spent time talking together. During one visit to James's home, Emily discovered that he had no money until the following weekend (5 days away) – he only had one Pot Noodle to last him for the whole week. After discussing this with James, Emily quickly liaised with the volunteer at the local church's food bank to see whether they could provide him with a bag of food. James was invited to the church and they reassured him that, if he was struggling to eat, he would be welcomed to collect a food parcel. James is now connected to his church and has met new friends.

Through that connection, and also connection with his local community café, a local volunteer offered to help by tidying James' garden, which he gratefully accepted. This helped him to maintain his tenancy and improved his relationship with his neighbours.

As the trust between James and Emily developed, during one particular visit, James confessed that he was in pain and showed his leg to Emily. His leg appeared to be heavily infected, inflamed and oozing. James said he had been to the GP a few weeks before, who had prescribed medication, but he had now completed the course. James explained that he was struggling to walk, had no means of transport and sometimes, due to drinking alcohol, could be forgetful. As a result, he had not been back to see his GP.

After some further conversations, James agreed that Emily could help him to contact his doctor to ask if more medication could be prescribed. Together, they telephoned the surgery and spoke with the doctor who agreed to prescribe a stronger antibiotic and stressed the need for James's leg to be dressed. Emily explained to the doctor that James was now unable to walk and asked if the district nurse could call to his home to apply a dressing. This was agreed and the district nurse visited James at home to apply clean dressings. Emily collected his prescription for him. James was very grateful and said "thanks for caring."

Without the contact with and support of Emily, it was inevitable that James would have been admitted to hospital if his leg had been left untreated.

Emily continued to walk alongside James for some time. Together they registered James with a GP surgery within a few minutes walking distance from his home. It would now be more accessible for James and easier for him to attend his health appointments.

Through getting to know the neighbourhood and local residents, Emily was able to support James to connect with his neighbours. One neighbour, Catherine, started to remind James to take his medication and keep an eye on him. She would remind James to attend his medical appointments to have his ulcers re-dressed. She also supported James to sort out his Department for Work and Pensions (DWP) pension as his payment plan had been changed. Another neighbour ran a local food bank and would check to see if James had enough food.

James was no longer isolated and was abstaining from drinking alcohol. Following his introduction to Emily, he has not called for an ambulance or been admitted to hospital. There were no longer concerns for his wellbeing; what had previously been regular safeguarding referrals and calls to the police had reduced to none.

James said that he had started to take some pride in his appearance and for the first time in a number of years had managed to save money and buy new clothes. He said he felt proud going into his local pub to have a meal. James has recently moved to a different neighbourhood; he has made new friends in his new community but stays in touch with his old neighbours, who still keep an eye on him. He remains abstinent from alcohol.

James continues to work with Emily, helping him to maintain his independence and delaying the time at which he may need to enter residential care.

61

James' world before introduction to Local Area Coordination

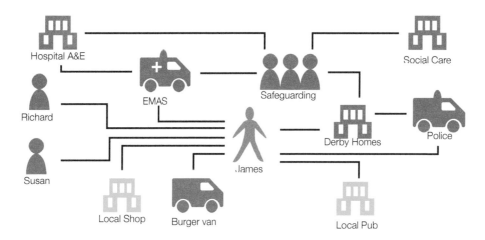

James' world after introduction to Local Area Coordination

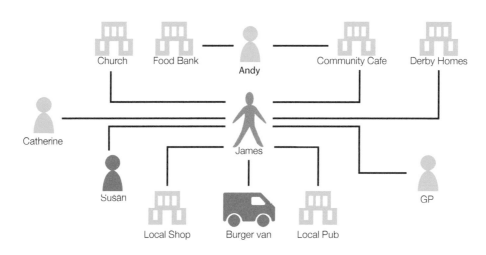

62

Change in James' quality of life

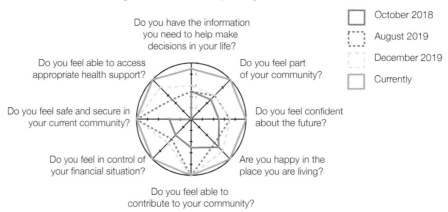

FIGURE 9. The impact of Local Area Coordination on James's life

4.4 Henry and Jess strengthen their relationship

by Catherine Viney

Henry and Jess met at a Day Support Programme and fell in love. Their parents, believing that they were not capable of understanding what being in a relationship meant, disowned them. With nowhere else to live, Jess and Henry made a camp in the bush out of town and made ends meet by taking out pay-day loans.

A few weeks after they set up camp, a bushfire threatened the area and they evacuated to a nearby free campground. Then it started raining. It was the most rain the area had in over 100 years. Their tent leaked and all their belongings became wet. Someone in their local community noticed this, and called the Local Area Coordinator, Camille, who lived and worked in the area.

Camille took the time to visit the campsite to meet Henry and Jess, get to know them and listened to their story. Henry and Jess really wanted a change of clothing and some warm bedding and so Camille introduced them to the local op shop (charity shop) owner. Camille also explored with them the things that were important to and important for them, and with Henry and Jess, prioritised where to start.

When Camille met them, she found that their living conditions were less than ideal with no access to running water, sanitation facilities, and cooking facilities. The tent was not in a formal campground and was not waterproof, and Henry's family had abandoned a broken-down vehicle with Henry's belongings in it. Jess had no belongings. They were under extreme financial stress due to taking out pay day loans to be able to purchase take away food.

Over the next 2 weeks, together, Henry, Jess and Camille explored local connections and solutions:

- The initial urgent response was to use a gift voucher to purchase some food
- Camille's contact in the local area said that they would be able to tow away the car
- Camille showed Henry and Jess where the local free campground facilities were
- They identified alternative accommodation, which led to a local member of the community offering a one-bedroom unit for them as a temporary solution. They have recently secured a rental flat in the open market
- Camille accessed some brokerage funding on Henry and Jess' behalf for a service provider to help them move, set up their new flat and immediately commence supporting them to live independently
- Introduced Henry and Jess to a community organisation who helped them put a plan together to manage their money and pay off their loans
- Connected Henry and Jess to people in their local community who could help them out from time to time
- Henry and Jess built confidence to let people help them, and get to know them better and have increasing control over their lives and decisions

63

As a result of receiving the support to build confidence and learn some basic living skills Henry and Jess, 12 months on:

- Are in a loving relationship, have their own flat and live independently, surrounded by strong friendships with people in their community
- They have paid off their loans and are saving for a holiday and hope one day to reconcile with their families
- Avoided the likely need for and use of formal residential and day supports, highly medicalised crisis services and unnecessary dependence on funded specialist services
- Have improved health and well-being
- Maintained and improved their choice and control over life decisions

64

4.5 Michelle works to make her family stronger

by Mary Flynn

In this piece, Mary, a Local Area Coordinator from Leicestershire UK tells the story of her relationship with Michelle who she met via a local resident who she had also been alongside. Michelle is a young mother with 3 children, 1 at school, 2 at home. When she met Mary, she was facing depression and debt and told Mary she thought she was a failure as a mother. Mary, tells the story from here:

Michelle was happy to meet with me and over a couple of visits shared with me her worries and her situation. We made a list of what she felt needed to do, and this helped her sort things into a priority of what to look at first. Whilst putting the list together Michelle also was able to talk about her mental health and how that impacted on her ability to cope day-to-day. She also accepted that she was avoiding facing her challenges, so things were getting worse. She had relied on her parents in the past to sort things out when things had got bad, but they were no longer in the position to do this.

We looked at the list together and Michelle decided that the first priorities were housing debt and her depression. She made an appointment to see her GP whilst I sat with her. Together we wrote down how she was feeling, for her to take to the GP appointment as Michelle finds it difficult to tell people about it. When the time came, Michelle was supported by her mother to attend the GP appointment. She also agreed for us to make a referral to a mental health service who were able to offer face to face talking therapy.

We then explored the housing debt. With her boyfriend moving back in the property Michelle's benefits had changed and with the expense of supporting another adult there had been a shortfall so they had chosen not to pay the Council Tax. We called the council together and with my support alongside her, Michelle was able to negotiate a payment plan to repay the debt. She was also happy for me to make an introduction to a service that would help with budgeting and ensure that the family were claiming all the benefits they were entitled to. We also completed a discretionary housing payment form to help cover the shortfall.

To help make the money go further I suggested that Michelle consider using her local food bank. Michelle was very resistant to this suggestion, as she felt that people would look down on her as her children only wanted to eat certain things. However, she said she was happy meet me at the food bank just to have a look and see how she felt. The visit went well, and she met a friend there so was more relaxed. Michelle joined the food bank and goes now when she needs too.

Michelle stuck to the plans we made, and she worked with both services around her debt and her mental health. We worked together to plan what she wanted her future to look like and the steps she would need to take and be able to take to get there. She planned her food shop and budget as well as activities with the children to make the day a bit more organised. This also gives her time to rest after work.

At our last meeting Michelle felt able to keep moving forward with less support from me. She felt more confident around her parenting and her planning skills. She knows that if she is struggling who to contact for help and she also knows that she is welcome to contact me anytime for either a quick pep talk or more support if more challenges arise.

65

I bumped into Michelle at the food bank a few weeks after our last meeting. She had walked down with her friend and was sat with a group enjoying a coffee – with a very rare smile on her face and she looks happier now.

Outcomes for Michelle and her family included:

- Increased control of money and better access to food
- Gained knowledge about informed decision making and budget planning
- Increased independence
- Connection with community and sustainable support

Outcomes for the community and services included prevention of need for other services and prevention of a crisis situation.

66

4.6 Carl goes from 'mental health service user' to citizen

by Anne Robinson

Anne, the Local Area Coordinator, was introduced to Carl by his GP as he was suffering from social anxiety, poor self-esteem and low moods. He found it difficult to engage with his family or peer groups and he spent his days at home. Carl lived with his partner and his young daughter but found interacting with his daughter especially difficult. He was estranged from his parents and sister. Carl was suffering from sleep apnoea, which had caused problems for him at work. As a result, he was off sick as he felt he was being subjected to bullying.

At Carl's request, Anne visited him at home. He wanted his partner to be there as he was nervous about meeting a stranger. He presented as a nervous but likeable young man who, once he relaxed, chatted easily. The first meeting was very emotional for Carl, as he spoke about his difficult childhood and his lack of contact with his parents and sister. Anne and Carl spoke about how life had been for him in happier times, and he said that his happiest time was when he worked in a bingo hall. He loved his job and had a close circle of friends. He desperately wanted to get back to having more confidence and getting out again.

Anne met with Carl on several occasions, just getting to know him and his family. This seemed especially important to gain Carl's trust before talking about what, if any changes he wanted to make in his life.

As their relationship developed Carl and Anne explored the idea of Carl attending a new Men's Support Group which was starting close to where he lived. Anne suggested they go along to the first meeting and, although nervous, Carl agreed to give it a go. Carl was initially very nervous, however, as the session progressed, he seemed to become more relaxed and willingly opened up to the group about how he felt and what he hoped to change in his life. When the members discussed how they saw the group developing and how to promote it, Carl voiced some excellent suggestions.

"Having you there made me feel confident. I was nervous but I knew that you would support me if people didn't like my ideas."

Carl bonded with one of the other men attending the group, Bert, who offered him a lift to future group meetings. Carl and Bert formed a strong friendship and often spoke outside of the group. The members had swapped telephone numbers on their first meeting and set up a WhatsApp group. Carl found this helpful as they were able to support each other when they were having down days. Carl also enjoyed the fact that he could support some of the others when they were struggling.

The group started to grow in numbers, and it was decided that a website be developed. Members voted on who would adopt roles and Carl was appointed the Mental Health First Aider. He sourced and attended a training course and gained a certificate in Mental Health First Aid. Carl also started to attend events to promote the group, conversing with professionals and members of the public with ease.

67

"I never would have thought I could do something like this. The thought of this before would have terrified me. I really enjoy having a role and I think I am really good at talking to people who are frightened or stressed."

Carl's health took a turn for the worse and he was admitted to hospital. During this time, he decided to make contact with his estranged family and they started to visit him. He confided in Anne that he loved spending time with his family again, but it was causing problems in his relationship. Sadly, his relationship broke down and Carl moved into a rented property next door to his parents.

Carl's only regret about leaving was that his partner was not allowing him to see his daughter and he felt a huge amount of guilt over this. Anne was able to give him information on different agencies who may be able to offer him help and support with this moving forward.

"I am happier now than I have felt in a long time. I just wish I could see my daughter but hopefully that will change in the future."

Carl's life had changed more than he could have ever imagined when Anne met him 16 months before. His role within the Men's Mental Health Support Group has changed and he is now in the process of taking over the running of the group. He has many ideas on how the group can develop and grow and is keen to hold some fundraising events in the future too. Carl has also secured a part time job in the local hospital and is awaiting a start date. His relationship with his family is stronger and they are able to support Carl when he needs it. Sadly, he still doesn't see his daughter, but has not given up hope that this could change in the future.

Anne's contact with Carl is less frequent now. She still occasionally checks in with him and he always calls her to update her on exciting changes in his life. It has been rewarding to watch Carl grow in confidence and make positive changes.

Outcomes for Carl included:

- Prevented things getting worse. Had Carl and Anne not met, he may not have had the confidence to take steps to change his situation
- Increased confidence which gave him the courage to explore his relationship and make bold decisions to improve his situation
- Moving closer to living his idea of a good life now. All that is missing is someone special to share it with and Carl feels he is now ready to start dating again

"I can't believe how my life has changed. I am happy with my life and am excited about the future. Thanks to you introducing me to the Men's Group, this was the start of my life changing."

68

4.7 Gemma works to get her child back

by Kim Harris

In early 2018, Gemma was finding life really difficult - her young son had recently been taken into foster care. Gemma only had a small support network; she was spending most of her time with her 'friend' and was taking on a lot of her responsibilities, such as helping with her children and paying for her family's food. Gemma was in a very low mood and had very little trust in professionals due to the way in which the removal of her son had been handled. She had her own flat but was not spending much time there and, most difficult for her, was allowed only very few hours contact with her son each week.

Shortly afterwards, Gemma met her neighbourhood's Local Area Coordinator, Sophie. Sophie spent time building a relationship with Gemma and her new partner. Gemma recalls that she wasn't expecting much from Sophie, having had numerous workers throughout her own childhood, part of which was spent in care; the workers changed regularly and she wasn't able to establish a connection with them. Then, when her own son was taken into care, she didn't feel supported at all. The biggest difference Gemma noticed in Sophie was how smiley and friendly she was. She immediately felt at ease.

Gemma and Sophie got to know each other and built a really strong relationship. Gemma was very clear about what she wanted to achieve; first and foremost, she wanted to regain full-time care of her son without the need for involvement from Children's Services. She wanted to move to a better home and also help to sort out her benefits.

Working towards these goals, and with support from Sophie, Gemma made significant changes in her life which resulted in her son being returned back to her full-time care. She felt that Sophie really earned her trust and knew that she could ask her advice without it being held against her.

Gemma's confidence has grown considerably, which she attributes to having Sophie alongside her for guidance and support. She commented, "Sophie thinks that [they're] just doing [their] job, but it's so much more". Things feel a lot more positive for Gemma and her family now. Her son is due to come off the Child in Need Plan, which will finish their involvement with Children's Services. When Gemma was expecting another baby, her midwife saw no need for involvement from Children's Services as she was considered to be very low risk.

Gemma has stopped having contact with people who she feels are not good for her; she now surrounds herself with people who are good for her and her children. She has good support from her son's nursery and they recognise the difference in Gemma. Once her new baby is old enough, she plans to return to work.

Gemma has moved with her children to a better home in a different part of the city. Even though she is now in a different neighbourhood, she keeps in touch with Sophie, sharing good news (and baby pictures), not just problems. Gemma no longer needs support from Local Area Coordination but knows that she can get in touch again should there be more things that she would like help to achieve.

69

Gemma's world before introduction to Local Area Coordination

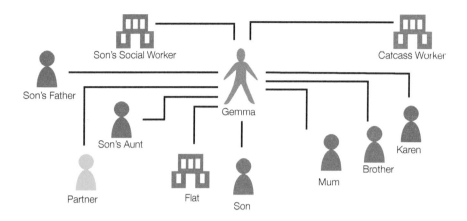

Gemma's world after introduction to Local Area Coordination

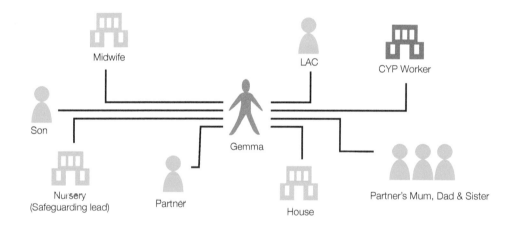

Changes in Gemma's quality of life

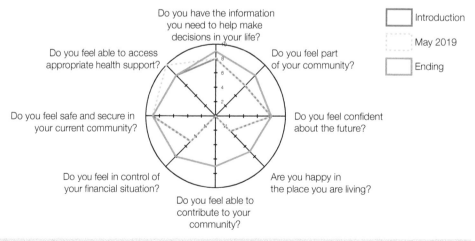

FIGURE 10. **The impact of Local Area Coordination on Gemma's life**

5. A leap of fact

From outputs to sustainable outcomes

Since its initial development in Western Australia in 1988, there has been an ongoing commitment to reflection, learning and improvement through research and evaluation. This has provided unique and ongoing opportunities to understand the long-term conditions of effective design, implementation, scaling and sustainability, that support (or obstruct) the full range of multi-level outcomes at individual, family, community and systems levels that Local Area Coordination offers.

Local Area Coordination evaluations have consistently shown that where there is strong, evidence and values-based design and strong, connected, contributing leadership, there are highly positive, consistent and sustainable outcomes at individual, family, community and systems levels. Where design is diluted, or there is a lack of effective leadership, outcomes are less positive and predictable.

Rather than just output focused measurements in evaluation, Local Area Coordination has placed greater emphasis on understanding of outcomes and how the Framework, role design and personal, local ways of working have impacted on individual, family, community and systems outcomes – 'what has happened, with whom, how and why?'

This is central in Local Area Coordination and is key to any effective human service and health evaluation.

'The question to evaluation then is not whether Local Area Coordination 'works', rather to unravel the 'black box' and deepen understanding of 'how' Local Area Coordination 'works' for people within a given set of circumstances and 'why' in order to identify the mechanisms of change and causation created through Local Area Coordination.'

Oatley (2016) p. 12

From the very beginnings in Western Australia and right through to more recent developments in England and Wales, regular, independent evaluation has helped highlight the purpose, design and expected outcomes of Local Area Coordination, as well as the contribution to local and national issues, challenges and policy direction. It has been the catalyst for reflection, ongoing improvement and growth through evidence. Interestingly, more traditional forms of service delivery have not had the same level of independent scrutiny during this period.

In this chapter, we will explore:

- The importance and value of ongoing reflection, learning and evaluation
- Key formative and summative Local Area Coordination evaluations and wider research
- Summary of evaluations so far and next steps and opportunities
- Two recent evaluations, methodologies and learning. Swansea University and University of Birmingham
- The outline of a planned multi-site evaluation in England

Why is learning and evaluation important?

Ongoing reflection, learning and evaluation is central to outcomes, sustainability, accountability and relevance. It helps us to understand what's working well or not so well, identify gaps and opportunities, stimulates innovation and informs future decision making and wider systems influence. It helps to identify and remedy 'programme drift', where design or practice has moved away from the core foundations, evidence base or values.

It is also central to understanding challenges and nurturing innovation and creativity, alternative approaches and possible partnerships.

Evaluation helps to:

- Understand what we have set out to do, how and why and then check to see if the design, implementation, behaviours and ways of working are doing this
- Find out what's going well and why: reinforce, repeat and grow conditions that support better outcomes
- Clearly identify where things are not going so well and why: set a clear action plan to remedy this and ensure accountability
- Identify gaps, obstacles and opportunities: embed flexibility, creativity and innovation
- Inform future decision-making processes, improve service design and make better use of resources
- Build understanding of external or other factors that affect outcomes: enablers and obstacles
- Safeguard individual rights

72

"This [resolving several issues faced by a person with significant interconnected challenges] would never have been done without the guidance, engagement and responsiveness of [the LCC and LCC local lead]. It worked seamlessly. Why the hell haven't we been doing that for years?"

Western Australia Department of Communities

Summary of Local Area Coordination evaluations

There have been over 40 Local Area Coordination studies and evaluations since 1988 including across Australia, New Zealand, Scotland, England, Wales and Ireland. Early formative evaluations in Western Australia focused on understanding the impact, outcomes and new opportunities of the design and implementation of Local Area Coordination alongside people with disabilities and their families in regional and rural communities.

These studies helped to reflect on 'What was working well and why?', gaps and opportunities for further development, wider reach and stronger outcomes. They showed that there were consistent, positive outcomes alongside people with disabilities, their families and the local community, as well as a multiplier effect from the financial investment.

Similarly, the involvement, leadership and decision making of local people (reflecting the diversity of people within those communities) in recruitment of Local Area Coordinators, in genuine partnership with the host organisation, also provides opportunities for multi-layered outcomes, including:

- Raising awareness of Local Area Coordination
- Increasing sense of community ownership, commitment and partnerships through the opportunity to actively contribute
- Increased knowledge of and connection with local people, communities, resources, opportunities and aspirations
- Building partnerships for change right from the start, before Local Area Coordinators even start their role, with individuals and families subsequently being part of evaluations, team meetings and training

This in turn led to exploring whether Local Area Coordination would also deliver similar outcomes and opportunities in urban and city locations, where early critics said 'this would never work in the city' because of the lack of community and the greater availability of services. An independent two-year study of metropolitan implementation across 10 sites, however, then clearly demonstrated the value of this approach in metropolitan and city settings with continued solid outcomes and high levels of consumer satisfaction. This evidence then provided increased momentum to move forward to scale.

Evaluation subsequently helped Local Area Coordination in Western Australia move from an 'innovation' to a core part of the state-wide service system and as a catalyst for wider system transformation (see Chapter 6, NDIS example).

The commitment to learning and improvement through research and evaluation led to further key studies, including:

73

- The *National Productivity Commission Report* (1998) of key reforms in government services delivery featured a case study on the Western Australian Local Area Coordination programme as a leading national reform. The report highlighted the core design, phasing of 'growth', consumer satisfaction and positive cost comparisons when compared with other services and states. It also identified reform outcomes and potential, through the development of social capital, effectiveness of choice and control through direct "consumer" funding, improved coordination of other services and sustainability
- A meta-evaluation (Chadbourne, 2002) looking at the quality, independence and fidelity of previous evaluations, as part of the Ministerial Review of Local Area Coordination
- A comprehensive 2003 Western Australia State Government Ministerial Review report highlighting Value for Money and the multiplier effect of investment, long term outcomes, "unanimous support in every key informant interview," operational challenges and the negative impact of layering "non-core LAC tasks"
- In 2010, Local Area Coordination received the Premier's *Award for Excellence in Public Sector Management* (Disability Services and Community). "The DSC's State-wide LAC programme has consistently achieved outstanding performance for many years and continues to provide innovative approaches to disability services that lead to long-term benefits" (Disability Services Minister, Simon O'Brien, 2011)

"Based upon measures of consumer satisfaction, family/carer satisfaction, consumer outcomes, service coverage, and cost effectiveness, LAC has proven to be a highly successful programme over an extended period of time. Successive evaluations, consumer satisfaction surveys and programme reviews have confirmed that LAC is a highly effective and contemporary support system for people with disabilities and their families."

Government of Western Australia (2003)

Local Area Coordination subsequently developed across Australian states and overseas, with varying degrees of design coherence and therefore outcomes. Again, where design was strong, there were strikingly similar outcomes, irrespective of location.

In Scotland, Local Area Coordination was introduced as a key recommendation of the review of learning disability services *The Same as You?* and progressively implemented from 2000.

"People deserve happier lives, not just better services."

Scottish Government (2008)

Subsequent reports and evaluations showed:

* The importance of a local, accessible, trusting relationships; quality of life improvements; family resilience; increased choice and control; better access to relevant information; valued opportunities and contribution in community life (Scottish Consortium on Learning Disability, 2006)
* Three main areas of achievement: a better overall quality of life for people; specific differences in individuals' lives; and particular areas, such as transitions to adulthood, where they believed they had made a wider impact (Stalker et al, 2007)
* Improved access to services, support and information
* Inter-agency cooperation was enhanced and increasing choice and flexibility in services for individuals and families
* Supporting individuals and families to build networks with each other
* Local Area Coordination was highly valued by individuals, families and staff from other agencies

"When I'm with my Local Area Coordinator, it's about me. My LAC understands how I am and helps me to do things for myself and be more independent. I have been able to go to places and try new things that I would never have done before I met my LAC. Everybody like me should be able to have a LAC."

Scottish Government (2008) p. 1

However, the 2007 Stalker et al. report also recommended the need for national guidance to inform a consistent approach to the development across Local Area Coordination in Scotland, with outcomes and sustainability being limited by variable understanding of Local Area Coordination at the system and operational levels that led to variable programme design, role design and outcomes.

74

*"There is wide variation in almost every aspect of the organisational
arrangements for LAC in Scotland. Some of this diversity indicates a departure
from the principles and ethos underlying the Australian model of LAC and was
experienced as problematic by many LACs."*

Stalker et al (2007)

Early conversations are now underway in parts of Scotland around exploring transition
to a consistent, national approach to Local Area Coordination, building on the current
international design and practice alongside people of all ages and all backgrounds within
local communities.

In New Zealand, a 2014 evaluation (Roorda et al) highlighted the positive experience of
people in terms of gaining or regaining control over their lives, decisions and choices and
the 'eight dimensions of value', reflecting core original Local Area Coordination Principles
from Western Australia and subsequent international developments.

*"Much of the value of local area coordination was evident in how disabled
people and whānau described their lives. Many respondents had experiences that
indicated they were now 'in charge' rather than having to fit in to someone else's
'agenda'. In telling their stories, the LAC's role was visible but not at the forefront,
indicating disabled people and whānau had strong ownership of decisions about
how they want to live their lives."*

Roorda et al (2014) p. 7

75

It is also highlighted the obstacles and limitations to wider change, outcomes and
sustainability. Rather than being embedded in both the system and community, creating
conditions for joint working, simplifying the system and better use of resources, it was
operating in parallel with, or as a 'tack on' to the existing system.

*"While Local Area Coordination remains in parallel with or as 'a tack on' to the
rest of the system, its take-up is likely to be variable. Local area coordination
will continue to be regarded as an 'optional extra' for some disabled people and
not others. Wider system changes are required in order for disabled people and
whānau to realise the full potential of Local Area Coordination. Local Area
Coordination cannot bring about the intended changes from the New Model of
inclusion, choice and self-determination for disabled people on its own."*

Roorda et al (2014) p. 7-8

As Local Area Coordination started to emerge in England and Wales, the previous learning was used to explore 'Is there any reason why Local Area Coordination would not equally benefit other people in local communities, beyond the original target group of people with disabilities in Western Australia and some limited work with people experiencing mental health challenges in Queensland and Stirling in Scotland?'

Local Area Coordination is now increasingly available more widely to people within participating local communities, built on this recurring cycle of progressive implementation and continuous evaluation. Subsequent international evaluations and reports have started to investigate, understand and analyse this broader reach of Local Area Coordination.

Access to food and medication	Leaving hospital
Agoraphobia	Leaving criminal justice
Anorexia	Leaving care (young adult)
Anxiety	Low self esteem
Asperger's	Mental health
Autism	Move to preferred living situation
Bereavement	Not in employment, education or training
Benefits and entitlements	Neglect
Family or carer support	Older age
Child carer	Parkinson's Disease
Community tension	Physical difficulties or disabilities
Dementia	Enforced prostitution
Domestic violence	PTSD
Drugs or alcohol dependency	School issues
Family related issue	Sensory impairment
Homelessness	Speaking up and self-advocacy
Housing issues	Stroke
Isolation and loneliness	Unemployment
Language barriers	Visual impairment
Learning or intellectual disability	Working with family member

76

TABLE 3. Examples of reasons for introductions

Evaluations have subsequently also started to more directly explore the mechanics of what makes Local Area Coordination work, why and how (Mason et al, 2021), the impact on individual, family and community resilience, relationship networks and mutual support, the value of intentional accessible early help and capacity building and wider financial (Roderick et al, 2016) and social benefits (MEL Research, 2016; Kingfishers, 2015 and 2016).

In Western Australia, a new evaluation (Department of Communities, 2021, unpublished) is showing emerging benefits across a broader population, including:

- Reach across culturally and linguistically diverse groups
- Child protection and family support services
- Delivering outcomes against Department Key Priorities
- Positive impact on individual and family confidence, connections, self-help, sense of control and contribution

Consistent with other international studies, they are also seeing reductions in:

- Presentation to medical services and emergency departments
- Police call outs
- Public housing tenancy dispute
- Isolation - increasing natural relationships and connections

See Figures 24 and 25 in the Appendix showing the breadth, reach and impact of Local Communities Coordination in Western Australia.

Connected and multiplier outcomes

The above evaluation also identified opportunities presented through a 'whole person' approach, rather than focusing on service aspects or deficits only.

"The evaluation found individual cases where a resolution in one area has brought about improvements in other areas. For example, supporting one person out of homelessness has had a profound and positive effect on mental health and in re-establishing connections to family and thus the natural supports that family can provide."

Western Australia Department of Communities (2021) p. 6

77

This isn't an accidental outcome, but an intentional part of design and practice as these outcomes are an expectation of Local Area Coordination. For every relationship alongside an individual or family, we would expect to see conditions emerging for multiple connected outcomes, as well as connected mutual benefits with communities and also with and between services. There have, and continue to be, strikingly similar, repeated outcomes in international evaluations where design, fidelity and leaderships are strong and maintained over time.

"People R-Outcomes surveys found statistically significant improvements in health status, health confidence and personal wellbeing for those receiving LAC support. These strong findings indicate LAC work is strongly welcomed and effective at changing people's general health status, health confidence and personal wellbeing."

Darnton et al (2018)

SYSTEM OUTCOMES (Reductions in)	CITIZEN OUTCOMES
Isolation and loneliness	Increased natural, supportive relationships
Visit to GP surgeries, medical services and emergency departments	Increasing community resources and connections
Referrals to Mental Health and Adult Social Services	Increasing mutual support in communities
Dependence on health, social care and housing services	Greater confidence in the future
Evictions and costs to housing	Better knowledge of / connection with local community resources
Public housing tenancy disputes	Improved access to relevant information, choice, control and self-direction
Safeguarding concerns	Improved health and well-being
Dependence on formal support and day services	Increasing control and self-care of own health
Anti-social behaviour and police call outs	Maintaining independence at home for longer
Financial benefit / value for money 4:1 (at 20% attribution)	Increasing access to volunteering, education, employment
Social return on investment 4:1	Avoiding crisis through early help
System wide 'prevention' and 'post service intervention' offer - prevent, delay, reduce	More able to build own resilience - needing services less
Less complex service pathways	Improved access to specialist supports

78

TABLE 4. Common system and individual, family, community outcomes (sourced from England, Wales, Scotland and Western Australia evaluations and reports)

This local, accessible support within communities, alongside the intentional work nurturing connections with and between local residents, supporting communities to identify and build new resources and the building of mutual support in local communities has been particularly important through the recent financial crisis and current COVID-19 pandemic. This will no doubt form part of future evaluations.

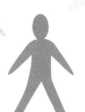

FIGURE 11. Feedback from people in Leicestershire, England, MEL Research (2016)

Highlights from a selected range of the growing number of international studies and reports since 1988 include the following:

1998: WA featured in Productivity Commission National Report - innovative approaches to the delivery of government services

- Importance of core design
- Phasing growth / expansion
- Positive comparisons / outcomes compared with other states
- Reform outcomes and potential

2002: Chenoweth & Stehlik, Queensland Evaluation - individuals, families and communities

- The 7 signposts (p. 6)
- Individual, family, community outcomes
- Early financial benefits
- LAC Objectives and performance (p. 73)
- Importance of safeguarding design and practice, especially in large bureaucracies

2002: Chadbourne, Edith Cowan University WA - meta evaluation

- Integrity of evaluation methodologies and consistency of findings

2003: WA Government - 15 year evaluation

- Showing long-term outcomes and growth
- Importance of role design fidelity
- Negative impact of adding 'non-core tasks' to the role
- Recommendations alongside indigenous, culturally and linguistically diverse communities
- High 'consumer' satisfaction and value for money

2003: Bartnik & Psaila-Savona, WA Government - value for money

- Framework for cost benefit
- Independent verification method of data
- National benchmarking
- Cost per person 35% lower than national level (p. 7)
- All key output areas had a higher level of consumer satisfaction than their national equivalents (p. 8)
- Preventive and multiplier effects of Local Area Coordination

2006: Scottish Consortium on Learning Disabilities - making connections

- Stories and feedback by individuals and families
- Impact of trusted, local support
- Individual, family outcomes

80

2007: Bartnik, Tamar Consulting - Australian Capital Territory Evaluation

- Very high level of support from individuals and families
- Good demonstration of a wide range of beneficial outcomes
- Challenges with developing and sustaining ongoing partnerships with service provides and the strategic interface with government as LAC is an externally contracted service

2007: Stalker et al - Evaluation of Scottish Executive Implementation in Scotland

- Better overall quality of life p. 2
- Key design and practice that create conditions for positive change
- Variability in design and practice impacted on consistency and measurability of outcomes
- Different contexts: rural settings, urban settings, across traditional service user groups
- Local Area Coordination highly valued by individuals, families and staff from other agencies, p. 6

2008: Scottish Government - National guidance on implementation

- Importance of national design consistency
- Financial benefit
- Individual, family, community outcomes
- How Local Area Coordination enhances self-direction and personalisation

2011: Fletcher & Associates - Middlesbrough First England Evaluation

- Formative evaluation
- People reported it made a difference to their lives
- Preventing people reaching crisis
- More effective partnership working with services
- A '1-stop' approach and holistic solution
- Helping reduce statutory service caseloads
- Supporting people other services 'find difficult' to support
- Cost effective
- Recommendations included: long-term funding and expansion, make part of 'front-end' of system

2014: Roorda et al - Evaluation of Local Area Coordination in New Zealand

- People feeling in charge of decisions about their own lives
- Eight dimensions of value
- Systems obstacles to LAC as a change agent

2015: Kingfishers Ltd - Social Return on Investment (SROI) in Derby, England

- 4:1 social benefit
- Recommends mainstreaming of community/person-centred approach to health and well-being
- High community impact
- Additional Council, Health, Fire and Police impact

81

2016: Roderick et al - Evaluation of Local Area Coordination across 3 localities in Western Bay, Wales

- Comparative study across 3 local authority areas
- Research involvement throughout design, development, inclusive community recruitment, implementation phases
- Key design factors
- Increasing inclusion and contribution
- Positive impact on isolation and natural relationships
- Financial benefit analysis and attribution

2016: Leicestershire County Council, England - Formative evaluation of Local area Coordination

- Financial benefit, avoiding critical incidents
- Positive SROI ration of £4.10 in accumulated benefit for every £1 spent
- Improved quality of life
- Reduced isolation
- Earlier positive preventative action
- Avoiding reliance on LAC / building individual capacity
- Increased choice and control
- Maintaining independence at home for longer

2018: Darnton et al - health evaluation, Isle of Wight, England

- Statistically significant improvements in health and well-being
- Positive impact on physical and mental health, community participation and happiness, resilience, self-advocacy, income, child protection and looking forward with future plans
- Prevention of worsening welfare

2019: Lunt & Bainbridge - City of York addressing isolation

- Summative evaluation
- Development of non-service solutions
  Preventative impact
- People able to upskill and volunteer
- People able to build positive vision for future
- Enable people to be heard
- Cost deferral
- Positive impact on community and system change

2020: Western Australian Department of Communities - Early formative evaluation

- Reach across culturally and linguistically diverse groups
- Positive impact alongside Child Protection and Family Support services
- Delivering outcomes against Department key priorities
- Impact on confidence, connections, self help, sense of control, contribution
- Reductions in: presentation to medical services and emergency departments, Police call outs, public housing tenancy disputes.
- Isolation - increasing natural relationships and connections

2021: Derby City Council, England - Evaluation 2018-20

- Relationships and community places, connections – reducing isolation
- Positive changes in quality of life
- Young people with experience of living in care
- Exploring wide system impact, including: reduced loss of tenancies, early discharge from Emergency Departments, reductions in care packages

2021: Mason et al, Southampton Solent University - Realist evaluation Isle of Wight, England

- Understanding what makes Local Area Coordination work, why and how
- The 'golden triangle' of listening, trust and time as key design and delivery factors driving outcomes.

82

"Stakeholders representing the formal service system identified individual cases where demand on their services has reduced and several expressed a view that the LCC was well placed to assist people so that they would not return."

Western Australia Department of Communities

The ongoing focus on inclusive, evidence-based learning, reflection, feedback and contribution, has been key in building the foundations for long term improvement, innovation, flexibility, accountability and relevance.

"Key positive outcomes for social workers through partnerships with Local Area Coordinators included having greater community knowledge, as well as releasing social workers to concentrate on supporting people with complex needs and issues, such as managing mental health crises."

Thurrock Council, England. Broad (2015) p. 43

Future opportunities

An ongoing commitment to review, reflect and improve all aspects of Local Area Coordination, from design and practice to leadership, will continue to support the evolution, relevance and impact of Local Area Coordination alongside local people and communities and to stimulate change within the service system.

With the increasing pressure on resources in health and human service systems, especially following the financial crisis (from 2008) and COVID-19 (2020/21), the focus on individual, family and community resilience and mutual support, reducing service dependency (or waiting for services) and understanding the conditions that enable that to happen are of greater importance than ever before.

Evaluation is a tool for learning, challenging, improving and influencing. It has the potential to stimulate change, influence policy and service design, improve practice alongside people and communities, drive and support evidence-based change. It also has the potential to drive better outcomes for people and communities, to ensure the voices of local people and communities are heard and to stimulate action for more personal, local, flexible, integrated services and to make better use of scarce resources.

New evaluations are underway in England (including a new multi-site evaluation starting in 2021) and in Western Australia. There are also plans underway for a 5-year summative evaluation of Local Area Coordination in Swansea and the first evaluation in Yishun Health, Singapore.

These will provide further rich learning to help guide us through a post-COVID-19 environment, understanding of the wider impact, reach and productivity on other services and contribute to reshaping the balance of use of diminishing resources between genuine capacity building and sustainable local solutions with the important role of specialist and funded supports and services.

Finally, in England and Wales, there is a connected 'network' of independent Local Area Coordination research partners, sharing learning, ideas, innovations and methodologies. We now have an opportunity to build international collaboration and learning partnerships.

83

Below are summaries of two key Local Area Coordination evaluations in England and Wales, plus an outline of the forthcoming multi-site evaluation in England.

- Innovation in Local Area Coordination research, written by Sian Roderick and Dr Gareth Davies from Swansea University.
- System transformation or just another service, written by Professor Jerry Tew and Dr Sandhya Duggal from University of Birmingham.
- New research on Local Area Coordination, written by Professor Joe Cook from University of Hull.

The Swansea University evaluation (Roderick et al, 2016) was, and continues to be, a key landmark in Local Area Coordination research and evaluation in the United Kingdom. It is unique, being the first to involve researchers in a fully immersive learning and evaluation process. This began at the early design phase (understanding the purpose, design, causal links between design/practice, outcomes and relevance to local and national challenges and policy), establishment of the integrated Leadership Group, observation of the inclusive community led recruitment process and subsequent implementation, training and delivery. It also moved forward understanding of measuring outcomes, especially around the impact on natural relationships (reducing isolation, increasing contribution) and financial and other benefits.

The Birmingham University evaluation explored how local authorities in England were responding to the requirement in the Care Act (2014), a key national policy driving reform of social care services, to prioritise capacity building and prevention in social care. This included two anonymised Local Area Coordination areas with different levels of design effectiveness, local understanding of Local Area Coordination and integrated leadership and resultant impact on outcomes and sustainability.

Finally, the third example is a planned, significant collaborative evaluation by Universities of Hull, Sheffield, Exeter, York and Leeds in partnership with the Local Area Coordination Network in England and Wales. The evaluation focus is on building an understanding of the contribution and transformative potential of capacity building programmes, like Local Area Coordination. It 'investigates how, why and under what circumstances Local Area Coordination can improve the lives of people open to adult social care whilst also reducing a need for statutory services in the first place.'

Local Area Coordination learning through evaluation continues to help improve, shape, create, adapt and maintain outcomes and relevance.

84

5.1 Innovation in Local Area Coordination research

by Sian Roderick and Dr Gareth Davies

The Swansea Local Area Coordination report provided the first formal feedback from the setup activities and initial activities. This early phase evaluation gave a particular focus to the emerging outcomes for individuals, coordinators and communities, as well as early indications of financial costs and benefits and the establishment of networks within communities. This work was intended to support both practitioners and leaders in optimising delivery, and policy makers in potential future use of Local Area Coordination.

Swansea is the second largest city in Wales and has a population of 241,000 projected to grow to 270,000 by 2036 with a disproportionate increase in the number of individuals aged 65 and over. It is also a diverse city with growing student and ethnic populations. While life expectancy by local authority may present broad averages of 75-80 years, the quality of life and life expectancy vary greatly from area to area within the city region with up to 23 years difference in healthy life expectancy between most and least deprived areas. The combination of health and socio-economic challenges within deprived areas has made them the focus for interventions including Communities First.

The ability to identify and reach all those with existing or (particularly in the case of preventative interventions) emerging needs is limited. At a UK level it is estimated that amongst older people there would be an additional 26% more 'service users' if 'moderate' needs were used as an eligibility threshold. This estimate was established at a time before eligibility criteria were tightened, further exacerbating the challenge of increasing need outside of council provision. This higher level of emerging demand and unmet need underlines the challenge faced within the region, and the importance of preventative actions that preserve valuable resources for those with greatest need.

Traditional approaches to health and social care across the UK and Wales continue to struggle to address growing demand, exacerbated by an ageing population, chronic disease and economic hardship. It is all set within a context of public sector austerity. The continued pressure upon public services makes it a challenge to embrace opportunities to adopt new practice, especially while maintaining quality and safeguarding obligations for services upon which users are highly dependent. This apparent paradox makes innovation most intriguing, particularly where further resource is unavailable, demand is growing, and change difficult.

These challenges, and efforts to address them are not unique to Wales. The Welsh Government, through the *Social Services Care and Wellbeing (Wales) Act 2014*, set new obligations upon organisations to work collaboratively in supporting individuals. The identification, appraisal, tailoring and adoption of relevant effective approaches to collaboration is itself a challenge for organisations balancing concurrent priorities. It is with this in mind that we were set the challenge of evaluating Swansea's implementation Local Area Coordination.

A formative evaluation undertaken by researchers at Swansea University commenced on 1st April 2015 and data capture began at the end of June 2015. Data collection continued through to April 2016.

85

Building the evaluation

The Swansea Local Area Coordination formative evaluation was developed between the commissioning partner, the Western Bay and Swansea University's Medical School (SUMS), and the Local Authority partners delivering the activity. We were researchers from the SUMS Enterprise & Innovation team and from the outset felt it important to work closely with Ralph Broad (Inclusive Neighbourhoods) to establish the ethos, values and a deeper understanding of the Local Area Coordination approach and gather expert insight into the development of our evaluation.

It was also important for us to understand the areas where Local Area Coordination differed from other services and initiatives. We were intrigued by the notion of a Local Area Coordinator embedding themselves into the local community and becoming a very accessible source of information and support based on the trust and organic connections they formed. By getting to know local people and forming these relationships, knowledge of resources and options grow. For individuals, families and the community itself, there are no eligibility or exclusion criteria, no time restrictions, no criteria or categorisation for help or support. It is a whole person and system approach that goes beyond meeting service needs.

During this year's pandemic, we have witnessed a highly effective and innovative response of Local Area Coordination to the communities it serves. Due to their relationships, knowledge and resourcefulness, Local Area Coordinators were able to mobilise and deploy sustainable natural community supports.

86

Evaluation design and methodology

The partnership approach to the evaluation was adopted to embed research, monitoring and evaluation into the Local Area Coordination activity, thereby allowing for a deeper insight into the work, whilst also making effective use of resources. The formative evaluation key components and aims were focused on:

- Assessment of project design and implementation
- Outcomes at the level of individuals, families, community and system
- Benchmarking of the processes and achievements of Local Area Coordination
- Recommendations for future development and expansion

As the Swansea Local Area Coordination implementation was still at a relatively early stage (given its long-term formula), our formative evaluation intended to support the development and implementation of the activity, and to lay a foundation for ongoing evaluation. To do this effectively, we felt that the data capture had to be not only address the cost-benefit (which was a main requirement of our evaluation) but also capture the true impact of Local Area Coordination on individuals, families and communities.

It was important to present the whole story and go beyond the numbers. The formative evaluation involved a number of approaches to data capture which contributed to developing more of a holistic picture of implementation Local Area Coordination in Swansea. The first step was to identify and engage with key stakeholders during development and the initial delivery. We interviewed key stakeholders at different stages to assess their expectations and involvement in the pilot, together with a mapping of their relationship with other actors.

This took us onto network mapping. Effectiveness of Local Area Coordination is dependent upon the successful engagement and tangible activity driven through individuals and organisations involved in delivering personalised support. A network and relationship science approach mapped the development and activity of Local Area Coordination across the network of individuals and organisations in working together towards common objectives.

The development of this was demonstrated across the regions in terms of linkages, activity and sustainability, all of which deemed important in realising the Local Area Coordination approach through an evidence-based design.

Understanding financial benefits

Using baseline data for costs avoided or incurred, the evaluation set out to determine financial impacts for the case studies. Beneficiary Case Studies were gathered for the purposes of scope of variation, the context, requirements, activity and outcomes. These were gathered through in-depth interviews with beneficiaries and those around them. These were then used to develop case studies from which impacts were assessed. With the addition of beneficiary interviews, an expert panel was gathered to review the development and implementation of Local Area Coordination. This consisted of senior social workers, health professionals and emergency service personnel.

In the first 3 areas within Swansea, during the early development-learning period (July 2015-April 2016) the report showed financial benefits of between £800k-1.2m (benefit cost ratio of between 2:1 and 3:1), based on most conservative assessments of expected benefits rising to between 3:1 to 4:1 when embedded within communities and partnerships established with services and partners. Only 20% of identified financial benefits were attributed to Local Area Coordination for this assessment – Local Area Coordination design and practice expects and celebrates effective joint working with people, families, communities, funded and statutory services. This is a positive outcome in itself.

Wider outcomes

The analysis and stories of change showed the significant value of walking alongside individuals, families and communities in a more personal, local, positive, flexible, human way, with people:

- Being more connected (less isolated) – family, friends, community
- Finding their own practical solutions, feeling more in control of their lives and decisions
- Needing services and formal support less
- More able to contribute – helping people to help themselves

It also showed:

- Positive impact alongside people from a wide variety of backgrounds and situations, in particular supporting people to overcome loneliness and isolation and alongside people facing very complex life situations
- Local Area Coordination 'tackling a broad range of social and personal issues'
- Local Area Coordination 'adding value across a range of public service pressures'

Design and partnerships

Since its inception in 1988, a wealth of expertise and experience amongst practitioners and researchers has been recorded, not least by Ralph Broad who supported the partnership during the implementation of Local Area Coordination in Swansea. We made use of this expertise to assess effectiveness of delivery at key stages through consultation and review drawing upon data collected through each of the research elements.

In order for us to gain a deeper understanding of the implementation of Local Area Coordination from within, we attended the recruitment process of the Coordinators. Through this immersive approach, we observed how community members were at the heart of the decision and the qualities (tangible and intangible) required in order to become a Coordinator. This citizen-centred recruitment approach provided immediate engagement and supported rapid development of both trust and progress.

After recruitment, we witnessed a 'springboard' effect where community members who were present at the interview greeted the successful candidates and made key introductions to important actors within the community. Members not only reported feeling valued for their contribution, but have remained engaged with the development of the programme in Swansea.

Therefore, during the interview process candidates were observed for their relational, listening, connecting, vision-building skills via the community conversations, as well as technical skills via panel interview. Successful candidates receive ongoing training, engage in regular reflective practice and work within supportive teams.

It is worth noting that Local Area Coordinators have a very low attrition rate, it is difficult to determine whether this is due to the nature of the recruitment process or the job itself. However, it is clear that Coordinators are exceptional at what they do. It is a multi-skilled role requiring beneficence and authenticity.

Embedding leadership

Previous evaluations of Local Area Coordination had shown the role of the leadership group to be integral to the successful sustainable progress of programme. Therefore, Swansea established a leadership group in March 2016.

As well as the researchers and the Local Area Coordination Implementation Manager, it consisted of Councillors and Cabinet Members providing a community perspective, representatives from social housing organisations, community voluntary services, the local health board, adult and child social services, prevention services, emergency

88

POWER AND CONNECTION | 5. A LEAP OF FACT

services, Public Health Wales and third sector organisations which include Citizen's Advice Bureau, Community Lives Consortium-supported living and services for people with learning disabilities.

Each member had their own perspective and different aspects of our findings focused the membership to the group, for example we found that isolation and loneliness was prolific in communities, this energised a particular agenda for one of the leadership group departments to address.

Through interviews and a facilitated workshop, we drew upon this group to define expectations, opportunities and challenges, and anticipated activities of the Local Area Coordinators. The group set 3, 6 and 12 month goals for the programme. They agreed that Local Area Coordination was a real opportunity for productive and collaborative local working within communities. The scarcity of resources was seen as a major challenge at the time, plus ensuring efficient use of resources and avoidance of duplication of effort.

Reflections

For many evaluations we are involved with, there is often a focus on the financial reporting and rightly so, however we felt it important to 'humanise' the figures by presenting qualitative elements into the report. These came in the form of short stories. We had a limited timeline and it was difficult getting ethical approval for all of the great stories we heard. However, the stories were impactful and added context and purpose to the investment.

For us as researchers, we were confident in the previous evidence which showed that Local Area Coordination as a concept could work and have significant impact for individuals, families and communities. However, it would need an effective leadership group to drive reform within the system itself, champion the programme, defend it against its harshest critics, and build a resilient and sustainable future. Throughout our research we observed what we termed as 'enablers' and 'obstacles'. Both can be useful to engage with for evaluation purposes.

Enablers were those who championed the programme throughout their networks and identified opportunities for shared value whereas 'obstacles' were considered temporary barriers to progress. Often this was due to the system and change behaviour or a lack of understanding about what Local Area Coordination actually is.

This prompted us to work with the Swansea Local Area Coordination team to organise one-day summit event at the University to share learning, generate ideas and discuss how to move Local Area Coordination beyond its implementation stage. From that event, it was clear that a shared vision is critical in driving the initiative forward. All involved, from organisations, to local people, families and communities, need a clear and coherent vision to create effective partnerships.

Shared vision should be predicated on a shared value to all involved, this has manifested itself in the generation of joint funding for Coordinators where both parties have experienced the benefits of prevention and being alongside those in need. Injections of funding into Local Area Coordination from Housing, emergency services and the public sector have all provided an intentional approach to building improved outcomes and whole system benefits.

89

A REPORT FROM THE CENTRE FOR WELFARE REFORM

Looking forward

In early 2021 we will once again revisit Local Area Coordination in Swansea and complete our summative evaluation. It will be interesting to see if our formative recommendations were absorbed into the programme.

Swansea has maintained fidelity of Local Area Coordination evidence-based design since the start. This is a testament to laying down strong roots at the outset. The programme has been successful in its growth and continues to expand its coverage. COVID-19 has presented unique challenges and we are keen to capture the learning and innovation generated by individuals, families, communities and indeed the system.

A new leadership team will need to be convened to support Local Area Coordination and enable it to meet the challenges as we rebuild our post-COVID-19 communities and reimagine a better way of working together.

90

5.2 System transformation

by Professor Jerry Tew and Dr Sandhya Duggal

Recent research has explored how local authorities in England were responding to the requirement in the Care Act to prioritise capacity building and prevention in social care (Tew et al, 2019). The Act recognised that carrying on with the previously dominant model (assessment for services and care management) too often delivered responses that were unhelpful – including provision of inappropriate services and (increasingly) using eligibility criteria as a way of just saying 'no'. The Act was not prescriptive in terms of how local authorities should achieve a shift towards a more upstream preventative approach and, perhaps unhelpfully, no ring-fenced funding was provided to support new initiatives.

While the first wave of local authority prevention initiatives tended to focus on introducing specific services such as re-ablement, assistive technology or signposting, some local authorities were aspiring to implement a more fundamental revisioning of the relationship between services and citizens, seeking to maximise social support and opportunities through working in more co-productive ways with individuals, families and communities. Typically, these second wave approaches involved:

- New forms of conversation and relationship between citizens, communities and service agencies: 'doing with' rather than 'doing to' or 'doing for'
- Facilitating new connections between individuals, families and communities in order to build or sustain social resources
- Finding 'smart' and non-bureaucratic ways of deploying relatively small sums of money 'upstream' so as to enable people to find solutions to their difficulties and to build effective support systems (Tew et al, 2019 p.5)

91

Within this context, Local Area Coordination offered a potentially powerful vehicle whereby local authorities could implement upstream preventative practice as required by the Care Act, and it could fit well with the aspirations of second wave approaches. Within the sample of local authorities that were studied in depth, two were implementing this, but in contrasting ways.

In Hanborough Local Area Coordination was introduced as an additional service to be piloted alongside existing services (essentially more of a 'first wave' approach) while, in Northshores, Local Area Coordination had been envisaged from the outset as the driver for a more fundamental second wave transformation of the ways in which the Council as a whole interacted with its citizens and communities. This very different contextualising of Local Area Coordination within the local service system would seem to have been key in terms of what subsequently transpired. Was Local Area Coordination central or an add-on?

In Hanborough, Local Area Coordination competed for space within a complex service field with apparently overlapping roles:

"We've funded a number of things and there's a lack of clarity, I think, about who's doing what and what's making the difference… A prime example of this is Local Area Coordinators would network with GPs, that would be part of the approach. But because we've invested in care navigators who are based in GP practices, receiving GP referrals, the Local Area Coordinators haven't stepped on those toes. So, they've diluted the potential offer."

Senior manager

In Northshores, there were some similar struggles in terms of establishing Local Area Coordination as a core approach in its own right, rather than something that just blended in with other more familiar approaches:

"People misunderstand Local Area Coordination, they think it's a kind of community connecting thing or they think it's social prescribing. You know, this is a way of working with very, very complex people who require very, very complex solutions sometimes."

Senior manager

However, there was greater clarity from senior leadership that Local Area Coordination should be a catalyst for wider system change:

"What we've done is we've learned lessons from Local Area Coordination which has allowed us to build on that approach… to think about systems and how we look at moving away from say that very much formal service support so how we can look at building more resources that are available in the community."

Senior manager

As long as Local Area Coordination could be seen as an 'add-on', it could be vulnerable; if it was designed in as the core of a wider system transformation, and it was seen to be enabling the emergence of more cohesive and 'can do' communities (with benefits beyond just adult social care), then its future was more assured:

"Everywhere in the council I go now people talk Local Area Coordination, whether it's at a leadership group where you've got planning and environment and you've got everybody in the room, everybody's seeing the benefit of Local Area Coordination, so the reward is huge."

Senior manager

A key issue that emerged from our interviews with Coordinators in both local authorities was how to maintain the distinctiveness of Local Area Coordination work rather than fall back on what may have been more personally or institutionally familiar, such as offering support or giving advice. Some Coordinators were good at articulating the 'subtle difference' between Local Area Coordination and the more 'doing to' or 'doing for' ethos that can characterise some other networking, support or social prescribing roles:

"My role is to get to know as many people as I can in order to find out what it is that the people want; what people have passion and enthusiasm for; not to do for them and not always support them as the more traditional services but to help them to take action on their thoughts and what's important to them. I think that's really the subtle difference but it's a really important one for what we're doing because if I step in to support people and take some of that ownership away or lead on some of it, it is actually not about them doing it themselves."

Coordinator

However, maintaining this distinctiveness was made harder in Hanborough by a perceived need to compete with other services, with credibility seeming to depend on delivering something familiar in conventional service terms. Nevertheless, this 'role drift' could be countered by having "really good supervision and peer support to talk about this… I've been very conscious to kind of try and do the lightest touch [but] I do slip into support worker mode sometimes" (Coordinator).

In Northshores, there was stronger support from senior management in maintaining Local Area Coordination distinctiveness and, crucially, creating reflective spaces (sometimes with external input) as a way of counterbalancing tendencies from within the local authority to revert to the norm of more conventional practice:

"It was a question of going back, are we being too true to those principles? Are we walking alongside? Are we making sure we do with and not to? Are we – you know – asset based in our approach? Do we have conversations? Are we getting sucked into bureaucracy? ….We sat down as a group and discussed those and identified ways in which that was beginning to happen and we kind of agreed to stop it from happening again."

Senior manager

93

A tension for Local Area Coordination in both local authorities was the extent to which it was owned in the community. In both, community representatives were involved in the recruitment process for Coordinators, but in Hanborough, this could be seen by the community as somewhat tokenistic, with no opportunity to have input in relation to the job description and shortlisting process. Feedback from community representatives indicated a disjunction between what the community wanted the Local Area Coordinator role to be and what it was in practice:

"The input I had was because I'm a community member and knew about various things, I was part of the interviewing process. Other than that, it was, 'Right, we're doing Local Area Coordination'. The Council decided that was going to happen."

Community member

In Northshores, Coordinators were more explicitly appointed on the basis of their values and commitment to the community - with local representatives being able to ask interview questions to test this out. However, there have remained some limitations in relation to effective community ownership of Local Area Coordination.

It has proved difficult to develop and sustain a stakeholder group of people who had accessed Local Area Coordination to provide challenge and support to the running and development of the service. Nevertheless, more informal networks have been involved in a more consultative capacity - including a Diversity Forum to focus on issues of inclusion, which was seen as particularly useful by one of our informants. From senior management, there was an acknowledgement that, although "whenever we do presentations or we're doing an event… we always involve them and they like to come along say what their experience", there was a need to involve them more effectively at a strategic level.

From this comparative evaluation, our key findings would indicate the importance of making Local Area Coordination central to a wider strategy for second wave whole system transformation, and for building in robust mechanisms for maintaining fidelity to the approach and substantive ownership of its development within the communities that it serves. Wider involvement and peer challenge through the national Local Area Coordination Network could be particularly valuable in achieving this. In the light of whether Local Area Coordination was seen as core to wider transformation, it was perhaps not surprising that a decision was taken by Hanborough not to continue the funding of Local Area Coordination – although some of the learning from the Local Area Coordination pilot is being used to inform subsequent approaches to developing community capacity building.

94

5.3 New Research on Local Area Coordination

by Professor Joe Cook

The Local Area Coordination Network and four of its member authorities (York, City and County of Swansea, Leicestershire and Derby) have won a new research grant with academics at the Universities of Hull, Sheffield, Exeter, York and Leeds. The National Institute for Health Research has funded the £321,272 project, led by the Professor Joe Cook at the University of Hull, for two years commencing in April 2021.

Understanding the contribution and transformative potential that capacity building programmes like Local Area Coordination can make to adult social care is vital. Although state and national evaluations of Local Area coordination have occurred in other countries such as Australia, New Zealand and Scotland, the evidence base that we have to work with in England and Wales is growing, though not yet comprehensive. This will be the first multi-site, summative and comparative evaluation for England and Wales.

This project is a unique collaboration between academics, the Local Area Coordination Network, Local Area Coordination managers, Local Area Coordinators, voluntary and community organisations and people who participate in Local Area Coordination. It investigates how, why and under what circumstances Local Area Coordination can improve the lives of people open to adult social care whilst also reducing a need for statutory services in the first place. It integrates qualitative life story methods with quantitative cost consequence analysis. This distinctive combination of methods will produce a more extensive examination of the effectiveness of Local Area Coordination; both in terms of its capacity to deliver benefits to the lives of people, their families (and the communities they live in) and as a preventive and capacity building approach.

The research methods are based on participatory action research approaches which prioritise working with professionals and communities and individuals in research and producing outcomes that benefit all partners not just academic knowledge. The involvement of people who participate in Local Area Coordination is embedded into the project; both through their membership on the advisory board and through our participatory action research approach which is focused on reflecting their voices.

The findings will be reported to the local authority partners and the Local Area Coordination Network at regular intervals and at the Local Area Coordination annual conferences and events. There will be an end of project report and conference as well as user friendly findings briefings. It is anticipated that at key stages interim findings will be released that inform both practice and policy; released periodically by the project partners.

We are really excited to start this collaboration and really looking forward to working with the four sites and with Nick Sinclair and the Network. This research would not have been possible without the support of the Local Area Coordination Network. We believe this is an ambitious programme of work with significant relevance to policy and practice. With increased emphasis on preventative and capacity building service approaches and Local Area Coordination programmes in the aftermath of COVID-19, this research will provide timely analytical findings to strengthen and inform policy in this field.

95

6. New developments

Ralph Broad (2015) previously reported on progress with Local Area Coordination in England and Wales, which for the first time included evidence from a targeted broader group from across social care, health, mental health and older persons. This development has continued in England and Wales with a number of new Local Authorities establishing Local Area Coordination sites and continuing this momentum. Examples of new established sites since 2015 include Wiltshire, London Borough of Waltham Forest, London Borough of Haringey, Kirklees, London Borough of Havering, City of York and Luton.

At the time of writing (March 2021), Isle of Man Government has now also confirmed the development of Local Area Coordination on the island, a welcome addition to the international network of Local Area Coordination areas. In Scotland, new national conversations are emerging exploring possibilities for transitioning from adult, disability specific Local Area Coordination to the emerging international focus across people of all ages, backgrounds and circumstances.

Since 2015, there have also been some significant additional learnings:

- New people – with the first expansion beyond disability in Australia as part of system transformation and integration (WA Department of Communities)
- New people – targeted cohort demonstration strategies including young people leaving state care and people attending Emergency departments (Derby City Council, England)
- New places – first full country expansion as part of the National Disability Insurance Scheme (Australia)
- New places – first demonstration planned in an Asian country (Singapore)
- New times - COVID-19 pandemic response and recovery (England and Wales)

A number of key points have strongly emerged from evidence gathered during this period. Firstly, the Derby City example is of importance because it demonstrates how a targeted cohort group can be embedded into a broad local area approach, rather than having a Local Area Coordinator for one target group only. This attention to fidelity of the broad Local Area Coordination framework and design we believe is outstanding as it preserves the strong local area connection which we know produces better results.

Secondly, as the evaluation results emerge from each new site, we again see the universality and consistency of outcomes where there has been a strong commitment to fidelity of design and implementation. Again, we have seen that core Local Area Coordination principles and strategies can adapt to new people, places and times.

Finally, through the example of the recent experience with the COVID-19 pandemic in England and Wales, the foundations of the Local Area Coordination practice framework and embedded connections to people and place have provided a strong foundation for developing personalised and local community-based support solutions for local people.

96

6.1 Western Australia moves beyond disability

by Tania Loosley–Smith

Western Australia has a population of 2.7 million people and is very city-centric. Nearly 80% of people live in the Perth metropolitan area, with the remainder spread over a vast area larger than Western Europe (2.65 million square kilometres). While ranking high on global liveability rankings, the State has significant variations in social and economic wellbeing. Aboriginal people in particular have poorer life outcomes and a history with government characterised by displacement and trauma.

The Department of Communities is WA's first multi-function human services agency, created in mid-2017 as part of a major reform of the Western Australian public sector. It bought together child protection and family support, housing, disability services, community services and regional services reform, most of which were formerly large standalone departments.

Transformation for better outcomes

Alongside the challenge of functionally integrating multiple agencies, 2018 heralded a unifying long-term agenda for the agency that focused on harnessing its breadth and scale to fundamentally change the outcomes for the State's most vulnerable people. There was a significant mood for transformational change and a recognition from staff that our whole was greater than the sum of our parts. The new agency's Purpose, Outcomes and Values reflected this aspiration:

97

"Our Purpose is about collaborating to enable pathways to individual, family and community wellbeing. And everything we do is about People, Place and Home and the deep connections between them."

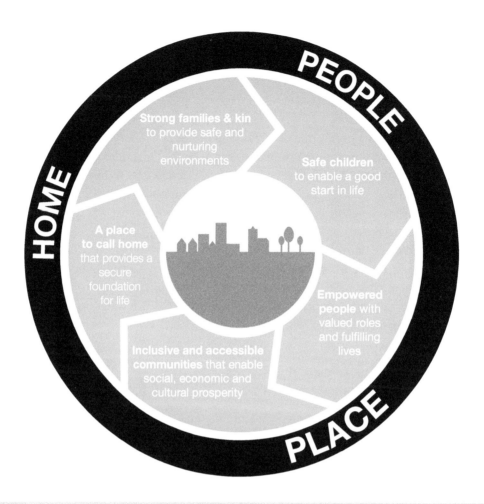

FIGURE 12. People, Place, Home – Western Australia Department of Communities

Search for new approaches to integrated support

This context also brought recognition that couldn't keep doing what we'd always done (i.e. more ambulances at the bottom of cliffs were not the answer; people needed new pathways to stop them going over the edge in the first place). So, some early reimagining of the current service delivery continuum brought a renewed focus on placed-based, person-centred, strengths-based and earlier support and solutions. These foundations had characterised the Disability Services system, but had largely been hollowed out of the broader Community Services system as it became more reactive and crisis driven. An appetite for serious systemic reform, increasing demand for core services (e.g. child protection, out of home care, social housing), and the strong evidence base from Local Area Coordination in WA Disability Services and the UK, provided fertile ground for Local Communities Coordination to emerge.

Part of the Local Communities Coordination value proposition was that it was a proven whole person, whole family, whole community and whole system approach, and uniquely positioned to help the new agency to:

- Learn about the needs and aspirations of people whose circumstances didn't neatly 'fit' one programme or agency or who fell through gaps
- Shift its reputation and relationship with communities from welfare intervention to wellbeing enablement
- Give visible life to a range of government priorities and structural reform aspirations through one initiative
- Push the reform boundaries beyond service collaboration and integration into a co-generative space where actions happen with and by community.

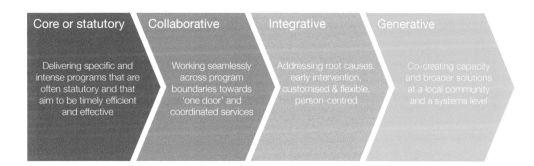

99

FIGURE 13. **An evolving human services approach - Western Australia Department of Communities, adapted from the American Public Human Services Association Toolkit**

The Approach

Local Communities Coordination was designed to test a new 'front end' to the new agency's service system. It aimed to provide a locally based, broadly skilled, 'go to' person to work earlier and more holistically alongside people to:

1. Find practical solutions to whole-of-life issues before they become insurmountable crises
2. Strengthen natural support systems and build capacity and resilience
3. Reduce cycles of dependence and demand on high-cost services

Our 'DNA' is all about working alongside people in the context of family, kin and community, respecting natural authority, and operating in an enabling rather than interventionist way. As a highly relational way of operating, Local Communities Coordination is strongly aligned with what Aboriginal people have been calling on government to 'be' and not just talk about.

Local Communities Coordination was formed around the following design principles:

- Better meets people's needs (whole-of-person and whole-of-life; individualised; one key contact; addresses causes not just consequences; focuses on natural supports not just funding and services; is a person not programme centred response; helps break cycles of demand and dependence)
- Supports government priorities (works effectively with vulnerable people of all ages and circumstances - e.g. Aboriginal people, families with young children, carers, youth, seniors, people with disability, people who are homelessness, women escaping family violence; people with mental health challenges etc)
- Financially responsible (reduces pressure on core services; over time will help rebalance our service model which is largely reactive rather than preventative)
- Delivers multiple outcomes (broad human service, not issue/cohort specific model; supports local service responses; multiple benefits across programmes and agencies, including Mental Health, Health, Education, Police, Justice)
- Built on 30-year evidence base from UK and WA Disability Services (proven track record)

Our approach promotes choice and control in the hands of people and communities and relies on a series of interrelated strategies: (1) getting to know people and what is important to them, (2) developing trusting relationships, (3) building natural networks and community supports prior to pursuing service or funding solutions, and (4) helping people to take practical actions to address aspirations and/or challenges in their lives.

Making it happen

Local Communities Coordination was approved by the agency's leadership in December 2018 as a two-year prototype in 7 regional and metropolitan locations. The first trial area went live in July 2019. Fittingly it was Albany (in the south west of the state) where Local Area Coordination was born in Disability Services way back in 1988. The other six country and metropolitan trial areas followed from July - October, giving us 25 operational staff in a variety of geographic and socio-economic locations.

Aside from the conducive reform and leadership context within the Department, the main things that allowed us to move so quickly were:

- Utilisation of experienced, values-aligned and locally respected and knowledgeable staff from the former Disability Services Commission
- Time upfront to talk with, and get buy-in from, colleagues and the community before taking introductions
- Input, training and mentoring from experts in the design and implementation of the approach (Eddie Bartnik and Ralph Broad)
- Small, agile project team based in the agency's strategy and transformation area with high drive and broad experience

Progress so far

While Local Communities Coordination is a medium-long term resilience effort, powerful impacts for people, communities and government are being seen early on. These include:

- Helping parents and carers who are overwhelmed and struggling to stay strong and care for their loved ones
- Supporting women and children as they rebuild their lives after leaving violent relationships
- Assisting people experiencing unstable housing or homelessness to access (or maintain) a range of housing options
- Helping people living with a disability or mental health condition to find the supports and services they need
- Helping people who are socially isolated to connect to family, friends, neighbours, peer or cultural groups that are important to them
- Providing information and connections that help people gain employment, maintain engagement with school, access childcare or support, resolve outstanding legal or court matters and secure needed services
- Reducing or preventing contact with high-cost services as the person is better able to manage or address underlying issues, e.g. police (less callouts), child protection (reducing risk of non-family placements), mental health and health (less use of acute medical and in-patient services), education (improved school attendance) and housing (addressing homelessness and reducing eviction risk).

101

We have assisted over 1,000 people in our first 12 months, the majority women, most with interrelated challenges and almost all experiencing social isolation. Survey and interview data along with a large amount of unsolicited feedback shows that Local Community Coordinators are highly valued and visible in their communities, something also reflected in the wide source of introductions (see Rishelle's story).

6.2 People leaving care or using emergency services

by Neil Woodhead

Over the course of the last 8 years, as the reputation of the Local Area Coordination team in Derby has grown. There have been a number of opportunities presented to us to secure additional funding to support the expansion of the team. More often than not these opportunities have been focused on a particular group of people who traditional services have had difficulty connecting with, or have what the system believes to be consistently poorer outcomes when compared with the rest of the population.

When considering these opportunities, we have learnt that it's essential to take the time to meet with the potential commissioner to try and figure out together, exactly what the problem is that they are trying to resolve. This really is time well spent as it then opens the dialogue to what Local Area Coordination really is and how it might be able to help make a difference. We have really used this time to clarify where both parties red lines are and establish if Local Area Coordination would be able to offer something into the mix… which invariably it can.

Often, these discussions are more to do with being clear about what Local Area Coordination is and isn't. What we will be prepared to do and what would compromise the approach. There have been a few instances over the years where we have walked away from potential opportunities as the request from the commissioner would have moved the team away from the core values and principles that make the approach successful.

The stumbling block tends to be about expectations around introducing assessments, data recording and a lack of understanding around what Local Area Coordination is. At times Local Area Coordination can seem too nebulous for potential commissioners but significant time has been spent honing how we record things alongside the people we support and developing information sharing processes with partners that allow us to demonstrate impact without Key Performance Indicators (KPIs) dominating the work.

Over recent years we have worked with two organisations who have seen the benefit of Local Area Coordination connecting with the people they find hardest to reach. They have worked closely with us to ensure that the commissioned work does not have a negative impact upon the delivery of the approach or the relationship development with the residents concerned.

In 2018 we were successful in our bid to the Department of Education's (DfE) Innovation Fund, where our work was focused upon young people with experience of the care system. In this case the there was an initial request to employ Local Area Coordinators who would only focus on the cohort identified, so they would only work with young people identified through the 'leaving care' criteria. However, by taking the time to build a relationship with everyone involved and by exploring the potential impact on outcomes we were able to reach an agreement that allowed us to recruit more Local Area Coordinators and extend the criteria of the whole team to include this group of young people.

This was the same approach we took in 2019, when we worked with our local Clinical Commissioning Group (CCG) to agree a specific piece of work around people the system described as being "high intensity users of services with chaotic lifestyles." As a team we were awarded the money for an additional post and we agreed to work with colleagues from our local Emergency Department to take introductions directly from that service and where possible prioritise these introductions.

One of the local innovations that came out of the DfE contract that went on to help us secure our CCG contract, has been our work we've been developing with people we're alongside and our partners around information sharing agreements. Once in place the agreement allows us to interrogate our partners data using anonymised codes to understand how often a resident used various services six months prior to their introduction to Local Area Coordination and then 6 months after. Allied to a strong history of qualitative data, this development has provided us with a persuasive argument for change.

Whilst in some ways picking up these types of contracts is frustrating given our belief that it should be an all-age locality wide, universal offer, it does allow for confidence from within the service system to grow. However, it also means that there is little certainty around sustainable funding stream; but that is the topic for another day.

What we already knew prior to picking up these bespoke pieces of work is that Local Area Coordination works. Where residents are isolated and without obvious connection to their own and their communities natural resources, introducing those individuals to a local community based worker, who isn't going to judge them or assess them but come alongside them and help them make sense of their own agenda, leads to better outcomes for all involved. Local Area Coordination is the best version of this.

"Young people reflected positively about their relationship with their Coordinator, which was often perceived as more accessible and reliable than other statutory provision."

Mollidor et al (2020) p. 6

The following graphic shows two very different, complex situations and journeys and reinforces that every person's life journey is unique to them. In both situations, each person reflects that the relationship of the Local Area Coordinator is highly valued.

103

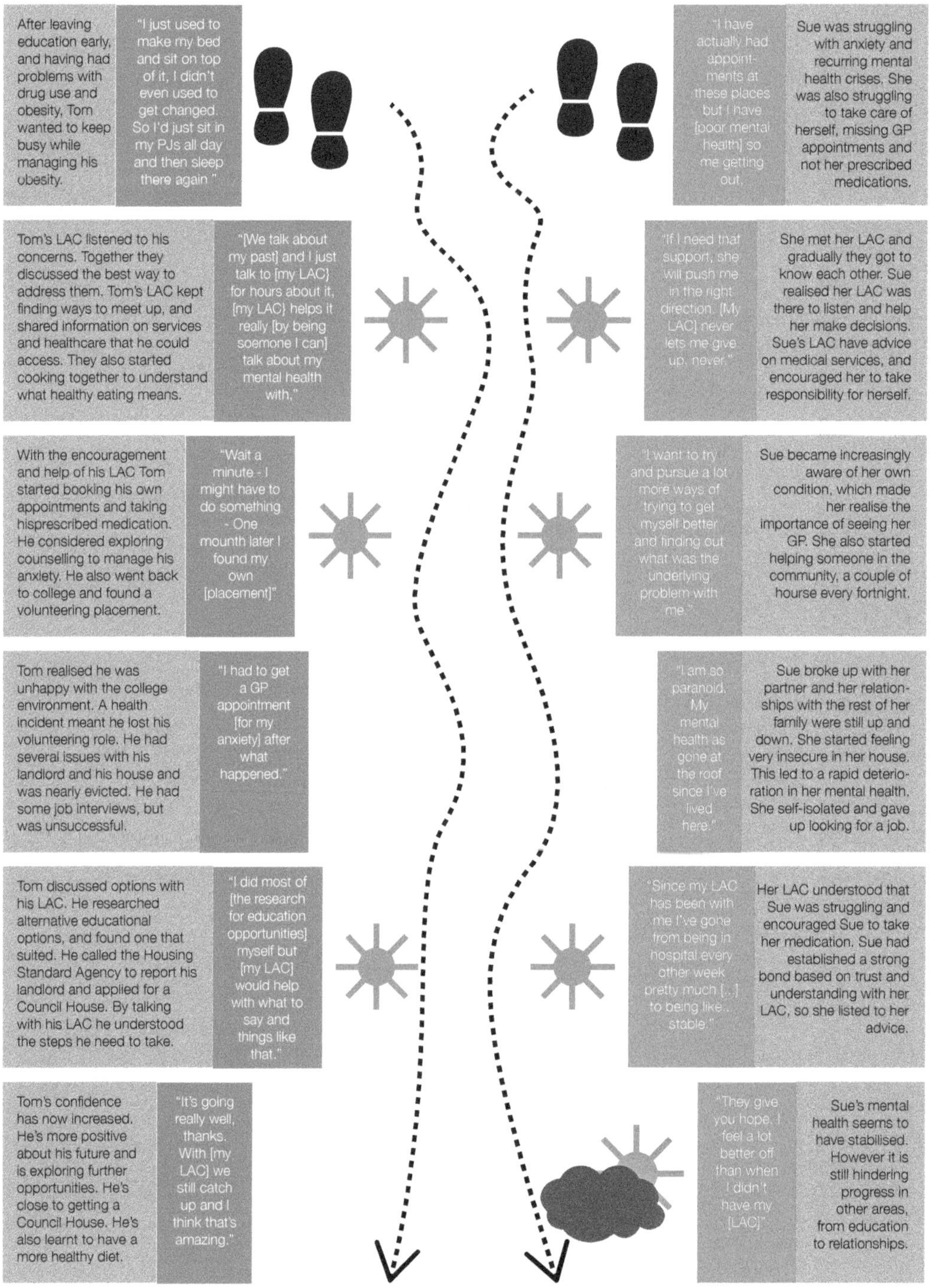

After leaving education early, and having had problems with drug use and obesity, Tom wanted to keep busy while managing his obesity.

"I just used to make my bed and sit on top of it, I didn't even used to get changed. So I'd just sit in my PJs all day and then sleep there again."

"I have actually had appointments at these places but I have [poor mental health] so me getting out.

Sue was struggling with anxiety and recurring mental health crises. She was also struggling to take care of herself, missing GP appointments and not her prescribed medications.

Tom's LAC listened to his concerns. Together they discussed the best way to address them. Tom's LAC kept finding ways to meet up, and shared information on services and healthcare that he could access. They also started cooking together to understand what healthy eating means.

"[We talk about my past] and I just talk to [my LAC] for hours about it, [my LAC] helps it really [by being someone I can] talk about my mental health with."

"If I need that support, she will push me in the right direction. [My LAC] never lets me give up, never."

She met her LAC and gradually they got to know each other. Sue realised her LAC was there to listen and help her make decisions. Sue's LAC have advice on medical services, and encouraged her to take responsibility for herself.

With the encouragement and help of his LAC Tom started booking his own appointments and taking hisprescribed medication. He considered exploring counselling to manage his anxiety. He also went back to college and found a volunteering placement.

"Wait a minute - I might have to do something - One mounth later I found my own [placement]"

"I want to try and pursue a lot more ways of trying to get myself better and finding out what was the underlying problem with me."

Sue became increasingly aware of her own condition, which made her realise the importance of seeing her GP. She also started helping someone in the community, a couple of hourse every fortnight.

104

Tom realised he was unhappy with the college environment. A health incident meant he lost his volunteering role. He had several issues with his landlord and his house and was nearly evicted. He had some job interviews, but was unsuccessful.

"I had to get a GP appointment [for my anxiety] after what happened."

"I am so paranoid. My mental health as gone at the roof since I've lived here."

Sue broke up with her partner and her relation-ships with the rest of her family were still up and down. She started feeling very insecure in her house. This led to a rapid deterio-ration in her mental health. She self-isolated and gave up looking for a job.

Tom discussed options with his LAC. He researched alternative educational options, and found one that suited. He called the Housing Standard Agency to report his landlord and applied for a Council House. By talking with his LAC he understood the steps he need to take.

"I did most of [the research for education opportunities] myself but [my LAC] would help with what to say and things like that."

"Since my LAC has been with me I've gone from being in hospital every other week pretty much [...] to being like... stable."

Her LAC understood that Sue was struggling and encouraged Sue to take her medication. Sue had established a strong bond based on trust and understanding with her LAC, so she listed to her advice.

Tom's confidence has now increased. He's more positive about his future and is exploring further opportunities. He's close to getting a Council House. He's also learnt to have a more healthy diet.

"It's going really well, thanks. With [my LAC] we still catch up and I think that's amazing."

"They give you hope. I feel a lot better off than when I didn't have my [LAC]"

Sue's mental health seems to have stabilised. However it is still hindering progress in other areas, from education to relationships.

FIGURE 14. Tom and Sue's Journeys

6.3 Full Country Expansion in Australia

by Eddie Bartnik

Australia is a country with a population in 2020 of 24.5m spread out over a land area of 7.7m Km2 which presents great diversity and many challenges. It does, however, also provide a unique example of continuous Local Area Coordination development from the original Local Area Coordination site in 1988 in Albany, Western Australia through to a complete national scheme from 2013.

From a single project in a rural area of Western Australia, successive expansions and evaluations led to complete coverage of the entire state over a 12-year period to 2000 and Local Area Coordination has remained a cornerstone of the disability system in that state since then, continually adapting to the changing environment. In particular, Local Area Coordination provided the original demonstration of personalised and localised support as well as direct consumer funding in the late 1980s. It was often described as a 'small scale lever of large-scale change' as the learnings from Local Area Coordination provided the evidence, confidence and stimulus to move almost the entire West Australian state funding for disability from a block system to an approach of personalised, localised support and individualised funding based on choice and control.

There were successive, smaller scale Local Area Coordination developments in some other Australian states and territories, notably Queensland, New South Wales, Australian Capital Territory and Tasmania. Despite several positive evaluations (e.g. Chenowyth and Stehlik,2001; Bartnik, 2007), none of these reached complete state wide scale nor achieved the critical mass and reform potential of the West Australian example (Bartnik and Chalmers, 2007).

In 2008, following a national report by the Australian government titled *Shut out: the experience of people with disabilities and their families in Australia*, and alongside a sustained period of collective and inclusive advocacy, the Commonwealth 2020 Summit in national parliament proposed a national disability insurance scheme. The Australian Productivity Commission is the Australian government's independent research and advisory body on a range of economic, social and environmental issues affecting the welfare of Australians, and in 2011 completed an *Inquiry into Disability Care and Support*. Specifically, they were asked "to undertake an inquiry into a National Disability Long-term Care and Support Scheme. The inquiry should assess the costs, cost effectiveness, benefits, and feasibility of such an approach" (p. v). In undertaking the Inquiry, the Commission was directed to "Examine a range of options and approaches, including international examples, for the provision of long-term care and support for people with severe or profound disability" (p. vi).

105

Search for a new approach

The Productivity Commission, further to a rigorous process of examining all the evidence, identified a range of core features of such a scheme – including "the inclusion of local area coordinators, disability support organisations and a wider community role for current not-for-profit specialised providers" (p. 36).

Their strong view was that "these core features would be best organised using a single agency — the National Disability Insurance Agency — that would oversee a coherent system for all Australians, regardless of their jurisdiction. The national model and its overseeing agency would learn from the best arrangements in place around Australia (such as local area coordinators in Western Australia and the accident schemes in Victoria, NSW and Tasmania)" (p. 37).

The value proposition to sustainability of the disability services system was clear – Local Area Coordination had a long track record of supporting people with disabilities and their families to build and pursue a good life in the community through building individual, family and community capacity. This results in outcomes at each of the levels of individual and family, local community and the service system overall as increased amounts of informal, community and mainstream support led to a more optimal use of funding and specialist disability services. Earlier studies by the Productivity Commission (1988) highlighted Local Area Coordination as a key national example of disability system reform and the West Australian government in their independent Ministerial review reported:

"Several external evaluations of both Local Area Coordination in Western Australia and elsewhere - most particularly Queensland - as well as internal evaluations and the value for money study that was commissioned as part of this Review, have confirmed that the Local Area Coordination approach provides value for money outcomes not matched by any other areas of disability service delivery. Further, the operational costs of Local Area Coordination have remained relatively stable over time, compared with other forms of service delivery. Compared with national benchmark data, Local Area Coordination provides more supports to more people, with a high level of satisfaction, at a cost that is more likely to be able to be afforded by Government."

WA Government (2003)

Implementation

In 2013, the National Disability Insurance Scheme Act was passed, establishing both the NDIS itself and also the National Disability Insurance Agency (NDIA). The NDIS itself is regarded as the biggest social policy reform in Australia since Medicare and the implementation of the new Scheme has taken place in a number of stages: Trial (from 2013), Transition (from 2016) and Full Scheme (from 2019). A fuller account of the Implementation of the NDIS is provided in the Productivity Commission Report on the Costs of the NDIS in 2017.

During the Trial phase, a number of differing approaches to Local Area Coordination were trialed involving differing combinations of planning, coordination and community focus as well as direct delivery or externally commissioned support.

To inform full scheme design, an internal NDIA review was conducted, which recommended the adoption of the long term Western Australian evidence-based approach of Local Area Coordination, subject to phasing in during the demanding transition period where over 400,000 participants would need to be brought into the Scheme from a wide range of federal, state and territory programmes, as well as those people not receiving a service.

106

Another key development in 2015 was the decision, due to the scale and complexity of the Transition period, to externally source Local Area Coordinators through a Partners in the Community model and contracted organisations, rather than as staff of the NDIA itself (NDIA, 2021).

Due to the incremental stages of the Transition period when individual states and territories signed their bilateral agreements, this led to a series of contracts with Partner organisations as each state and territory came on board. The contract specifications outlined the role, key activities, broad geographical areas and performance metrics of Local Area Coordinators. However, the tender process and contracts did not require Partners to implement the role in a connected, localised manner. So as with some other countries such as Scotland, there have emerged differing implementation approaches to the evidence-based role and ongoing challenges in bringing the role back to a nationally consistent level of quality and consistency.

Although not specifically reported by the National Disability Insurance Agency, in 2020 it has been estimated by the NDIA that there are more than 3,000 Local Area Coordinators in the NDIS employed through the 13 Partners in the Community organisations, supporting a significant proportion of the 412,500 NDIS participants as well as a broader population of people with disabilities through the Information, Linkages and Capacity Building (ILC) strategy. In addition to the Local Area Coordination role, other key NDIS staffing groups include NDIS Planners, Early Childhood Early Intervention (ECEI) Partners in the Community and a small number of Community Connectors for particular hard to reach target groups.

The NDIA provides a national public Quarterly Report with the September 30th 2020 report outlining 100% national geographical coverage with approximately 412,500 participants, satisfaction ratings around the 84% and progress on participant and carer outcomes. Significant transformation has occurred and it is certainly a work in progress as the Scheme starts to mature in a full scheme environment.

107

Challenges

The rapid growth of Local Area Coordination nationally as part of the NDIS has provided many benefits to the participants of the Scheme and the broader Australia community as Local Area Coordinators have played a key role in building the NDIS to this point. National data on the Scheme as a whole is reported by the NDIA and individual Partners collect and provide key data and evaluations as part of their contractual and quality arrangements.

There are, however, a number of key challenges ahead, including differing understandings of what 'good' looks like in Local Area Coordination, the availability of a suitable workforce, reorienting the role back from the initial focus on planning and funding during transition, and need for a national network approach and technical support to build greater consistency across the 13 partner organisations.

Firstly, due to the differing starting contexts in each state and territory, people across the country came to the NDIS with differing understandings and experiences of Local Area Coordination. For example, in Western Australia, Local Area Coordinators were a household name with decades of credibility, whereas in Victoria for example and a number of other states, there was no experience to start with or any existing Local Area Coordinators on the ground. For the 64,000 people with a psychosocial disability estimated to come into the NDIS from the health system, they had no experience of choice and control of their funding let alone knowledge of what a Local Area Coordinator could do. The NDIS started with a wide range of very uneven starting points across the country and differing bases of trained and capable staff in each jurisdiction ready to step into these new and sometimes previously unknown roles.

Secondly, the pressure of Transition and fixed bilateral targets to bring people into the scheme, created a focus on participant numbers and getting their individual funding and plans operating so that people could access much needed supports. Early training was also focused on bringing people into the NDIS versus the broader and more holistic Local Area Coordination role. The time is right for a strong reorientation back to the strengths of family, friends, community and mainstream services within people's plans and a rebalancing of the strong Transition period focus on individual funding arrangements. The 2020 NDIA review of the Local Area Coordination Framework is very welcome as Local Area Coordinators can make an increasingly vital contribution to better lives for people with disabilities and their families and overall scheme sustainability.

Thirdly, the consistency and quality of Local Area Coordination support nationally is a major challenge for the Partners in the Community approach with delivery through 13 different organisations. Finding the right form of a national network approach to collaboration, training and development, whilst working in a contract environment of competitive tenders, requires additional safeguards compared to a direct delivery approach.

108

6.4 First demonstration in Asia, Singapore

by Dr Wong Sweet Fun

In June 2010, Khoo Teck Puat Hospital (KTPH) was opened to serve more than 550,000 people living in the north of Singapore. It was the first hospital to be built in 10 years and was sited in the heart of the neighbourhood. The healthcare landscape and pressures (Wong, 2018 and Design Singapore Council, 2020) at that time warranted a data-driven design-led population health approach to create lean systemic and sustainable change to the improvement or maintenance of residents' health.

Residents saw the hospital as the default option for any health issues, contributing to access bottlenecks. Working daily with sick patients in a clinical environment, it was easy to forget that residents were assets in their community. Once we discharged them, they were out of sight, out of mind, and replaced by other sick patients who needed our care. That care became our primary driver as we strengthened care coordination and developed a variety of excellent healthcare services. Community support services were expensive and created further reliance on the healthcare system. Patient behaviour seemed complex and unintelligible until we considered that the majority of healthcare takes place in the low acuity setting of the communities and homes of people, and outcomes are dependent on their daily lifestyle choices. We thought of medical advances as improving our aim at shooting a target, but the situation was really more akin to hurling a bird at the bullseye. It would save us much effort to first understand what motivates and attracts (Design Singapore Council, 2020) the bird to the end point instead (Elby, 2015).

We learnt avidly from global best practices and moved away from the idea that health is solely delivered by the healthcare industry. A good healthcare system takes pride in its citizens' good health, rather than just of its excellent healthcare services. Our language changed from a needs-based vocabulary to strengths-based, from 'doing to and for' to 'doing with and by' as we learnt to 'don't just do something, stand there.' We leveraged Singapore's unique housing and neighbourhood planning to introduce Asset-Based Community Development (ABCD) in 2014 and community-led self-management eco-systems parallel to the participatory city concept within seven years.

Outside of the hospital, at various infrastructural amenities and touchpoints, residents look out for each other's health at the Wellness Kampungs (Centre for Liveable Cities, 2019) and during Share a Pot® (iF World Design Guide, 2017) gatherings. Community Nurse Posts are within walking distance from homes, providing basic health advice and screening. Recovered patients now have more avenues to be active, happy and contributing members of their community. Residents also begin to see the healthcare system as a safety net instead of a cure-all.

BUILDING ECOSYSTEMS

A Culture of Self-Help

Any group activity is an opportunity to include everyone and encourage bonding. Any physical activity anywhere to improve physical function is better than none.

By being as inclusive as possible and allowing residents to participate to the extent that they are comfortable and able, we can help to shape a culture of self-help and build resilient communities.

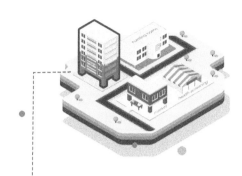

110

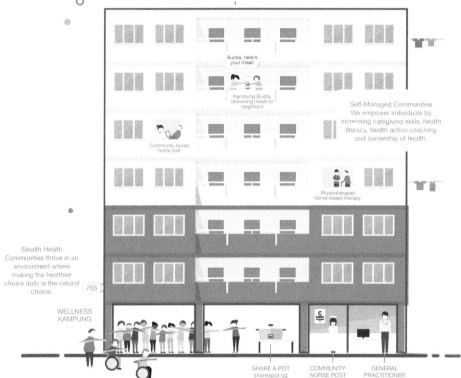

Self-Managed Communities
We empower individuals by increasing caregiving skills, health literacy, health action coaching and ownership of health.

Stealth Health
Communities thrive in an environment where making the healthier choice daily is the natural choice.

Staying Healthy Together
Through activities that bring them together, residents to form networks of mutual support.

Visible Access
Community partnerships and mass outreach initiatives bring health closer to home.

FIGURE 15. Community-based self-management eco-systems – Singapore, Yishun Health

ECOSYSTEM DEVELOPMENT PRINCIPLES

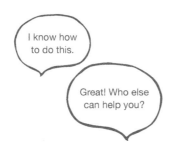

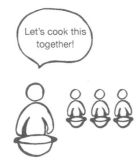

1   Facilitator, not provider

2   Focus on action that creates behavioural change

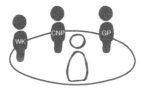

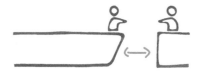

3   Individually good, even better as a team

4   Delivery to the last mile

111

FIGURE 16. Ecosystem development principles – Singapore, Yishun Health

Over 80% of Singaporeans live in public high-rise apartments organised around local amenities for daily necessities. At the ground floor (void deck) of such apartment blocks, residents can drop in at the Wellness Kampung, Share a Pot® or Community Nurse Post. Medical needs are attended to by nearby general practitioners who run their private clinics.

How will Local Area Coordination fit our Singapore context?

Singapore has enjoyed a stable majority government that has created conditions to formulate and implement long-lasting and reliable whole-of-government policies around housing, health, education, security, social integration, national development, defence and trade over the past 55 years.

Local Area Coordination supports people with disabilities, mental health needs, older people, sick persons and their families to achieve their vision for a good life, to be part of and contribute to their communities, and to strengthen the capacity of communities to be inclusive. The language and philosophy of self-direction, self-management and self-determination matches what we need to pull all our developmental pieces into a coherent community self-management eco-system. It starts with building valued, trusting relationships with individuals, families and communities, then opening up positive conversations about their gifts, skills, aspirations and connections. Services are the last part of the conversation, but are sometimes needed, along with the know-how to access, navigate, choose and manage these services.

In a major reorganisation of Singapore's public healthcare system in 2017, Alexandra Health System, which run KTPH and Yishun Community Hospital, merged with the National Healthcare Group (NHG) to form an integrated healthcare cluster, upscaling best practices and optimising resources for healthcare delivery to more than 2 million citizens within the central region of Singapore.

Aligning to NHG's Community Nursing model to Sense, Care, Coordinate and Strengthen, Local Area Coordination can work in concert with community nurses, anchor community partners and Asset-Based Community Development (ABCD) practitioners to strengthen the community capability and capacity in its accountability to self, belonging to each other and care for the whole. In the north, we identified 9 sites covering approximately 95,000 residents where the principles and practice of Local Area Coordination and ABCD could be rolled out.

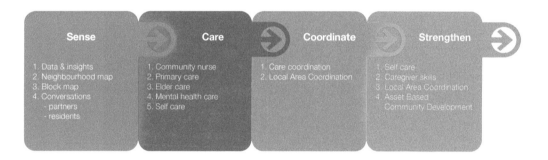

FIGURE 17. Local Area Coordination as part of a Community Nursing Framework - how Local Area Coordination and ABCD work together for better supported self-management in the community setting - Singapore, Yishun Health

A 'reverse cold call' to the Local Area Coordination Network led to our propitious introduction to Ralph Broad in February 2018. NHG made an opportunistic study visit to Derby on 22 May 2018, where Neil Woodhead and the then LAC Network CEO Samantha Clark had organised a memorable community meet-up with local area coordinators and members of the Derby City Council with our Group Chief Executive Officer and key NHG leaders. In a hectic week in October 2018, Ralph visited Singapore and presented a plenary lecture at the Singapore Health & Biomedical Conference (SHBC) attended by 3,500 participants, conducted a masterclass for NHG administrators, allied health and clinical staff, and did a whirlwind tour of our community eco-system.

Two teams made multi-site deep dive studies of integrated community care models (including Local Area Coordination, ABCD, Participatory City, Year of Care) to London, Thurrock, Barking & Dagenham, Croydon, Swansea, Frome, Trowbridge, Newcastle,

Leeds and the Isle of Wight in March and November 2019. The generous sharing by the Local Area Coordination Network and communities has helped us to clarify what Local Area Coordination is and is not and has demonstrated the many ways that health-social integration can be contextualised in local communities and cultures.

Since 2019, we have continued to work directly with Ralph, and are poised to involve some naturally connected residents to initiate a community-led Local Area Coordinator recruitment. We train our staff for effective strengths-based 'first conversations', not for information-gathering assessments to fit inclusion criteria for services. In parallel, we direct programme resources towards resilience and sustainability specifically in the areas of induction, training, partnerships, community knowledge and connections, for continued long term outcomes. These bring us closer to better lifelong care and aim to achieve the quadruple aims of improved residents experience of care, better population health, reduced per capita cost of care and sustained care team wellbeing.

Orchestrating community transformation for better population health management and improvement is indeed challenging. We were fortunate to learn and adopt and adapt successful global concepts and philosophies. Now to pull it all together, watch it grow, and spread the word. There is still much to do - it's not going to be easy, but it's going to be worth it.

I would like to thank the following for their collective work in driving Local Area Coordination development in NHG: Evon CHUA Yiwen, WOO Wan Ling, THAM Sinma, NG Tzer Wee, TAY Choo Yian, NG Huoy Ling, ONG Wei Wei, LOW Beng Hoi, Bastari IRWAN. I would also like to thank Claire OOI Wen Yu and Albert FOO for their contribution to this manuscript.

113

6.5 Getting started in Yishun, Singapore

by Evon CHUA and WOO Wan Ling

Developed in the 1980s, Yishun is a residential town located in the north of Singapore and home to over 220,000 working-class Singaporeans. As a health system, Yishun Health has data to show that the northern population struggles with poor health at a younger age, but years of working alongside the community have also shown us many of its strengths and successes. We have discovered stay-at-home mothers who organise food distribution to care for their neighbours, older residents who lead morning exercises in their neighbourhoods to start the day bright, and young people who step up voluntarily to be trained as local first responders in their blocks. There is so much possibility in this community that can be built upon.

Building our confidence

Our journey of distilling the design process with Ralph Broad began in 2018. We have learnt much from our collective visits to local area coordinators, leaders and residents from Derby, Thurrock, Swansea, Wiltshire and Isle of Wight. The learnings from these visits helped us understand the nuance of building and restoring supportive relationships for people living through difficult times. In the past 18 months working directly with Ralph, we deep dived into the operations, implementation processes, supervision and evaluation tools, and contextualised their successes and challenges in order to adapt Local Area Coordination to Singapore.

We invested in conversations to ensure that our multidisciplinary team of nurses, allied health professionals and administrators began with the right practice language. We lined up training to introduce Motivational Interviewing, Asset-Based Community Development (ABCD), Year of Care and Local Area Coordination to build up our repertoire of strengths-based conversational skills across professional functions. The Year of Care is about improving care for people with long-term conditions (LTCs) in the National Health Service (NHS). It is about putting people with LTCs such as diabetes firmly in the driving seat of their care and supports them to self-manage. It transforms the annual review into a constructive and meaningful dialogue between the healthcare professional and the person living with long-term condition.

Through these sessions, we gained a deeper appreciation of the value of a good life conversation and the change that Local Area Coordination could offer to our system.

Building connections with stakeholders

We learnt about the importance of stakeholder engagement from decision makers and other care partners in the initial development phase and shared our learning with stakeholders from the health, social and community care sectors. Together, we envisaged the positive change that Local Area Coordination could bring to our care ecosystem. This early engagement generated excitement and sealed the commitment from our local partners to give the Local Area Coordination implementation a good chance of success.

114

Currently, we count two regional hospitals and a local network for seniors as our key stakeholders. We hope that this energy generated can be harnessed to form a Local Area Coordination Network in Singapore in the near future.

The next step we took was to identify the areas for implementation. Based on our local population data and the spread of existing service and community partners in the region, we divided the implementation into three key development phases for the next four years. Identifying the specific areas for implementation made it easy to invite local residents from each of the neighbourhoods to participate in the hiring of our coordinators. Planning ahead and prioritising the neighbourhoods also allowed us to manage and pace the reviews of our progress with our leadership and management.

Building on knowledge

We adopted the practice philosophy of Local Area Coordination into our everyday work and changed the way we worked with individual residents. In-depth exchanges with our residents gave us powerful local stories that helped with the understanding and appreciation of Local Area Coordination locally. These experiences will add value as case studies for future supervision sessions and learning sessions with our teams.

Our strengths-based training and early Local Area Coordination encounters also help to dispel early hesitation about translating Local Area Coordination culturally in Singapore. Our experience reinforces the core of Local Area Coordination – the value of individual gifts, skills and assets, the powerful and positive role of families and relationships in our lives, and the contribution that local communities can make as alternatives to professional health and social care services. It reflects a basic humanistic, yet universal and profound, way of working alongside people whose lives have been overcrowded with services.

115

Building on COVID-19

The COVID-19 restrictions pushed us to be creative with our recruitment plans. The involvement of our local residents was not something that we wanted to compromise, so recruitment plans had to be delayed by three months. Thankfully, locally transmitted cases in Singapore were brought under control by June 2020, making it possible for us to plan for a small group of residents to join us on-site as panelists for the Citizen-Led Recruitment.

The applicants were invited to a Candidate Open Day on Zoom. The session was created to let candidates clarify their understanding of Local Area Coordination, allow us an opportunity to prepare the candidates better, and curate an interview session that would be beneficial to both the residents and the candidates. The Citizen-Led Recruitment was held across two of our Wellness Kampung with safe distancing guidelines in place. Hosting the sessions online meant that candidates had to explore the use of technology to interact with the residents. They did not disappoint, and we were treated to videos, interactive slide shows and engaging presentations that the residents enjoyed. At the end of the tiring six-hour long Citizen-Led Recruitment, we could still feel the pulse of the energy in the room from both the residents and the candidates – and it was one of enthusiasm and hopefulness.

COVID-19 may be the biggest challenge of our generation (thus far), but it also reminds us that the core of human services is to build and form valued relationships between individuals, families and communities. Services should be brought in only at the last part of the conversation. Even as the COVID-19 situation comes under control in Singapore, the economic, social, public and individual health impact will continue to endure for many more months. We are glad that as we move into recovery in 2021, our residents will be joined by our first group of Connectors, chosen by them. We are excited to move into a new phase of our implementation journey and look forward to having meaningful conversations on 'what is strong, and what matters' with our residents as part of our new normal.

There were many times during our design and implementation phase where we considered taking shortcuts to speed up our implementation. Despite the challenges, we were glad that every step of the process, however arduous, had successfully created space to the strengthen the capacity of our communities to welcome, value and include each other.

116

6.6 Local Area Coordination and COVID-19

by Nick Sinclair

In early March of 2020, it became clear that normal life as we knew it was about shift significantly as a result of a growing outbreak of COVID-19 which had already had devastating effect in other parts of the world. When the UK national lockdown was announced on the 23rd of March 2020, plans to adapt and flex Local Area Coordination to meet the personal, community and systemic challenges on the horizon were already underway. Likewise, the Local Area Coordination Network (which leads the development of the approach across England and Wales), quickly pivoted too, ramping up our learning, sharing and connecting functions in new and innovative ways. Our members started to regularly gather online in order to connect, share learning and raise each other's spirits during what was an exhausting and demoralising time for all. Our Network began carefully documenting the learning coming back from Local Area Coordinators and other sources including the emerging government guidance and policy. This allowed us to form a live COVID-19 Crisis timeline (through the lens of Local Area Coordination) which has been documented for reflective practice and posterity.

In the immediate days of the lockdown and being temporarily unable to walk alongside people in the community as they normally would, Local Area Coordinators were tasked with supporting their local community and council-led efforts to respond where needed most. The Councils in our Network used this opportunity to build on the strengths of the Local Area Coordinator skill set, ensuring they were able to support in ways that played to their existing relationships, skills and community connections. Coordinators carried on working, albeit in many cases remotely, with people they were alongside before the lockdown as many of those people were already disconnected from their neighbours and local services for whatever reason. In addition, many Coordinators took on temporary new tasks within health and social care, including running some type of virtual community hubs, making welfare calls and taking introductions from colleagues running call centres, etc. All this change and focus on vulnerability was a major test on the values and principles of Local Area Coordination, but it was one that Coordinators rose to with great passion and spirit.

Reflecting on this challenge of focusing on strengths during a time of crisis, the table below (created from a contribution for this report via Kathryn Humpston a Derby Local Area Coordinator), highlights how Coordinators were still able to respond with creativity, sensitivity and a deeper interest of the bigger picture of someone's vision for a good life. The snippets below are of citizens of the community Kathryn serves, calling up the local hub she was running for help. We have included here what we think a likely traditional service response could have looked like, compared with the actual Local Area Coordination response led by Kathryn. Names and details have been anonymised.

117

PERSON CALLING THE HUB	A TRADITIONAL SERVICE RESPONSE	LOCAL AREA COORDINATION RESPONSE & ACTUAL OUTCOMES
Betty, in her 80s, telephoned the hub requesting a befriending service.	Signpost Betty to befriending service (if one available) and tell her to call back if things get worse.	Kathryn supported Betty to make regular contact and build friendships with 5 of her neighbours
Brian telephoned Adult Social Care requesting a formal support package to help with his shopping.	Signpost Brian to front door for Adult social care assessment to take place some weeks later (if at all). The assessment would likely lead to a non-eligibility outcome.	Brian and Kathryn had a conversation and he was connected with a neighbour, Michael, who visits twice a week to fetch his shopping and checks on him to see if he is ok. They have become good friends. This has prevented a need for Adult Social care assessment and support.
Sarah calls up struggling with mental health concerns.	Signpost Sarah to a mental health support service or give phone numbers for crisis team if things get worse.	Sarah was supported to become a neighbour who would collect prescriptions for her older neighbours. She says this has given her a purpose and reduced her feelings of loneliness.

Social value created in the community and prevention of mental health crisis for Sarah. |
| Janet, in her 80s, contacts Hub for help with collecting her medication after having shielded for 4 months. | Number given for medication collection and delivery service. | Connection made to medication collection and delivery service. However, following a good life conversation, Janet is now making a contribution by sewing face masks for her neighbourhood. |

TABLE 6. Focusing on strengths and relationships during a time of crisis

Where safe, many Local Area Coordinators continued to work in the community supporting the connectivity of Mutual Aid group efforts and ensuring food and medicine distribution efforts ran smoothly for those who were shielding etc. The work Coordinators had supported historically around building community capacity to be self-supporting, welcoming and caring places proved essential in inspiring and encouraging a community led COVID-19 response. These existing relationships also ensured those responses were not lost in the mix of increasingly 'higher level' planning but rather they have become the cornerstone of those local government led plans. This was aided by the fact that Coordinators had a foot both within the communities they served and within their local service land. The expansion of Local Area Coordination in Swansea during the pandemic was directly based on the evidence of the value they were providing in those areas already covered. People in existing Local Area Coordination areas were better prepared and connected when COVID-19 hit plus supportive neighbours and communities were quickly mobilised.

This is neatly reflected in the following example from Swansea provided by Local Area Coordinator Emma Shears who writes:

My role began in November 2017 in the Cwmbwrla Ward and Gendros, from this time I have been building positive relationships with people of these communities. Gaining knowledge and connections with individuals, families, local councillors, associations, groups, faith groups, organisations, businesses and service partners. From this, I have been able to introduce local people, organisations and groups to each other, resulting in many further relationships and the formation of Cwmbwrla Community Events (CCE).

CCE became key in the response to the pandemic, and when lockdown began the positive connections already in place enabled community-led action and an immediate local response. With mutual support amongst its people and Local Area Coordination being present, this set the foundations to enable people to support one another.

Collectively this community helped people facing extreme challenges, such as: loss and bereavement, employment changes, job losses, ill-health, mental health difficulties, learning difficulties, pregnancy and birth, single parents with low income, families with low income, asylum seeker communities, people with a visual impairment, disability, as well as those shielding specifically for their safety. The community helped by setting-up the following:

- A local Emergency Food Resource specific for people's nutritional and dietary needs (funded by Western Power)
- A WhatsApp group – for coordination of requests (prescription collection, food shopping, welfare checks, etc.) and for communication between the people helping
- A Facebook page – to circulate up-to-date coronavirus information

119

As well as connections already in place, new relationships formed and together this allowed for innovation, creativity and collaboration. In quick response, the following was also established:

- A weekly community newsletter (delivered to those isolated and shielding),
- A book-bundle sharing scheme (to lift spirits and aid connection),
- A local Treasure Hunt (helping to keep families and children entertained), and
- The making of a local book through listening and collecting the stories of personal history within the community, enabling conversations and connections to grow. (Jones, 2020)

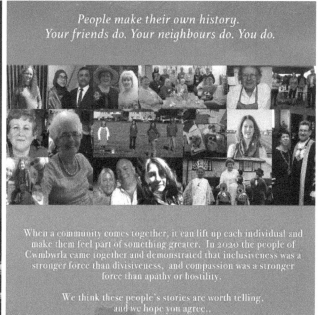

FIGURE 18. Circling the square – local community celebration, action and mutual support through COVID-19, with Local Area Coordination support

Being a single point of contact and being easily accessible has ensured a focused and sustainable community response during coronavirus. New skills and passions have developed as a result with people looking into future possibilities of Cwmbwrla Community Events and the new connections made.

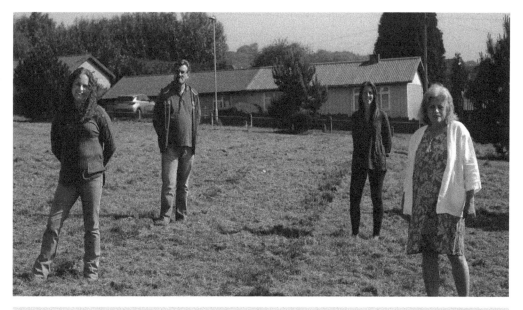

FIGURE 19. Seren Aldron, Peter Black, Emma Shears, Amina Jamal from Cwmbwrla, Swansea

"If it wasn't for Local Area Coordination I wouldn't have known where to go to offer my help. Thank you for giving me the chance to be a good neighbour, Cwmbwrla now feels like home and I have made great friends from this experience, it has changed my life for the better."

David Jones, Community Member

As we write now (September 2020), Local Area Coordination in England and Wales is becoming central to local recovery, rebuilding and renewal efforts with a recognition of community power being central to emerging plans where it operates. Coordinators are exploring with people they are alongside how they may continue to connect in the post-COVID-19 world, including continuing online connections and meetings which have seemingly grown in value and preference for many people. It has been particularly encouraging to see new areas in England and Wales getting in contact with us to explore how Local Area Coordination may make the difference where they are. This reflects a growing post-COVID-19 recognition of the need for a new deal between citizens, communities and local statutory institutions. The Local Area Coordination Network remains proudly in place in order to convene, champion the approach and support the development of it at every opportunity.

"Throughout the COVID-19 pandemic, our team of Local Area Coordinators have demonstrated just how valuable they are. In York, they were already well established in their communities with plenty of local connections, which were just what was needed to be able to respond to the many issues they met. 'Walking alongside' residents to support them to solve problems themselves, [they] saved precious time for specialist services, enabling efforts to be focused on those in greatest need. In many cases, some low-level help was exactly what was needed to stop small problems getting bigger, and that's what Local Area Coordinators really do well. Hard working, flexible, adaptable and kind, Local Area coordinators are just what is needed to help bring our divided society back together again."

121

Councillor Carol Runciman, City of York Executive Member for Adult Social Care and Health and Chair of York Health and Wellbeing Board

7. Leadership development

This Chapter highlights the need for collective and inclusive leadership to initiate and sustain Local Area Coordination and demonstrates some of the key fidelity and sustainability features outlined above, namely:

- Nationally shared values and Local Area Coordination Framework, regular connections through a Network with international best practice connections
- Deliberate investment in leadership, new ideas and partnerships
- Within and cross-sector leadership, creative resourcing involving a combination of recycled and new resources as well as pooled funding from different silos

The four case studies that follow demonstrate key examples at local, national and international levels:

- The England and Wales Local Area Coordination Network, founded by Ralph Broad in 2015 and written with the current Director Nick Sinclair
- The International Initiative for Disability Leadership, written by their International Lead Eddie Bartnik
- Swansea's Leadership Group written by Councillor Mark Child
- A new social contract between citizens and state, written by Professor Donna Hall, Chair of New Local in the UK

122

7.1 The England and Wales LAC Network

by Ralph Broad and Nick Sinclair

This is a combined account of the early formative days of the Network from Ralph Broad as founder, along with the perspectives of the current Director Nick Sinclair, demonstrating the evolution and sustainability of this unique member-funded network.

The idea of the Local Area Coordination Network was born out of a commitment to embedding Local Area Coordination principles, values and evidence in everything we do, at every level and with all of our relationships – the importance of 'programme cohesion' leading to sustainable outcomes and people and community-led change.

As we started the Local Area Coordination journey in England and Wales in 2008, we sought to understand and explore the conditions in Western Australia that contributed to long term, outcomes and sustainability. Building on Ralph's early shared support to some national developments in Scotland, the connection with Eddie Bartnik was pivotal in building our early foundations for getting started and for what would become the Network in the future.

Eddie gave his time to help with 'unpacking' the thinking, practice and possibilities of Local Area Coordination, accessing useful resources, building connections with colleagues in Western Australia and leading the early Local Area Coordination introductory workshops in the North East of England in 2008-09, with the great support of Paul Davies, the Department of Health North East Valuing People Support Team Lead. These conversations led directly to Middlesbrough moving forward as the first Local Area Coordination site in England. Most importantly during this time, we were able to 'take time' to explore, build connections, form a plan and take the first steps of building authentic, values and evidence based Local Area Coordination in a new country and context and start to think about the conditions for successful implementation, scaling and longer-term sustainability.

When reflecting on some of the key 'building blocks' in Western Australia that supported outcomes and sustainability, a number of things became obvious. These included the significant value of having overarching national leadership, a shared national Framework (including shared vision and design), an intentional culture of mutual support and collaboration between areas, space to explore and be curious and an ongoing commitment to evaluation, shared learning and evolution. The issue then became: 'How do we achieve these same core foundations and conditions for fidelity, outcomes and sustainability in a different location, with different, separate service and governance structures?' The idea emerged of an intentional Network of participating areas committed to strong design, leadership, learning and ongoing positive change and evolution. It has since created a rich resource of learning, mutual support, positive challenge and supports the ongoing development of Local Area Coordination alongside people, families, communities and the wider system. The Network builds the conditions for learning, strength, consistency, growth and sustainability.

In hindsight, the obvious question now would be 'Why on earth would we not want a network of collaboration, learning and improvement?' The absence of shared vision, principles and design increases the risks of the dreaded 'postcode lottery' where any innovation or service may mean different things in different places and lose its original

123

purpose and outcomes. This, in turn, leads to people and families experiencing significant variability in the type and level of access, support, opportunities and outcomes and reduces the wider opportunities for person and community driven change. Suddenly, there would be the risk of a well-intentioned service being an obstacle to citizenship, embedding inequality and quickly losing relevance.

To get started, the Local Area Coordination Network for England and Wales was established within Inclusive Neighbourhoods, where informal connections and conversations of mutual support and shared learning between emerging Local Area Coordination areas, including Derby City, Thurrock, Swansea and Isle of Wight, started to grow. We then worked together to explore the desired purpose, value, actions, opportunities and outcomes of a connected national Network. The first Network Newsletter was shared in March 2012, introducing Local Area Coordinators, sharing learning and stories from areas, sharing core information about Local Area Coordination and welcoming contributions from innovators leading complementary strengths-based work elsewhere.

We then started to build:

- Opportunities for Local Area Coordinators from different regions to meet, get to know each other, share stories, and access new learning and reflection
- Meetings for Local Area Coordination managers to connect, work together to build shared resources, problem solve, share ideas and build a consistent approach to information gathering for learning, monitoring and evaluation – the cycle of learning and improvement
- Senior leader gatherings to explore the strategic value of Local Area Coordination, share learning and build a network of support
- Connections between emerging research partners – a network of research partners
- The first two England and Wales Local Area Coordination conferences

A key decision at the outset was to invite Eddie Bartnik to be first Patron of the Local Area Coordination Network. This built on our original collaboration and maintained a direct link with the original (and ongoing) Western Australia development and the long history of learning from across Australia and subsequent international developments. Eddie also played a key role in early Network learning and development sessions with managers and senior leaders, supporting the development of effective evaluation approaches, contributed to our national Local Area Coordination conferences and building connections with, and participation in, IIDL Leadership Exchanges.

As we have learned, gathered significant evidence and grown, this ongoing relationship has also resulted in Inclusive Neighbourhoods and the Network being invited to contribute to international conversations and conferences, sharing the new learning from England and Wales. The opportunity to move from being a receiver of support to being a contributor.

As the number of councils adopting Local Area Coordination in England and Wales grew, so did the emerging Network of various people passionately leading it in their local authority area. It was clear that there was both appetite and an imperative for collaboration. So, in 2015 the Network formed a stand-alone Community Interest Company (CIC) with supportive, visionary leaders Sian Lockwood and Alex Fox as founding Board members and Samantha Clark as the first Director. In 2018, it then found a strategic home as part of Community Catalysts CIC. Community Catalysts has proven

124

to be a great home with synergy across its existing programme of work, with a remit and scope that has widened significantly as a result.

The Local Area Coordination Network is the home of and lead agency for Local Area Coordination in England and Wales. Its members recognise the importance of working together and having a central repository for Local Area Coordination knowledge and best practice. It develops in a way that mirrors the principles, design and behaviours of Local Area Coordination around the value of relationships, mutual support, vision building etc. The founding Network leaders carefully designed it upon the principles of the Local Area Coordination itself, for instance those of 'working together', 'contribution', 'lifelong learning' and 'community'. The leadership of these principles was fundamental to the successful development of the Network and remain so today. Taking this approach to the Network has been be particularly important given that each site is led by an independent local authority. It has become a positive and powerful voice for growth, development and wider reform in the UK.

In line with the original intent, there now continue to be a number of sub-networks within the Network, including one for operational managers, senior leaders, coordinators and elected members (politicians) of the councils leading Local Area Coordination. The Network is also supported by a number of research partners from different universities and bodies who have led local evaluations and are keen to share and reflect upon learning. It has dedicated staff resources (funded through membership fees) to help it convene and who regularly facilitate training, gatherings and conference events as part of a wider programme of strategic work. Members attend regular gatherings both in the community and online, passionately opening up their own learning, experience and resources to each other's shared endeavour. They also offer peer support to each other to tackle common challenges, building upon the shared vision, principles and values with new learning and evidence that is emerging all the time. A major focus of the Network's programme is on supporting each other to stay true to the principles and fidelity of design, ensuring Local Area Coordination is not pulled back into the status quo of the system and instead begins to have the opposite effect over time.

125

In December 2020, the Local Area Coordination Network held its first ever 'Local Area Coordination Week' in an attempt to raise the profile of the approach both locally where it is happening and in new potential areas too. The week included events such as an online conference focusing on ten reflections on the guiding principles of Local Area Coordination from some great supporters of the work. It also included the first ever attempt at a 'global gathering' with Local Area Coordination people from all parts of the world coming together online to explore key themes and issues, not least the potential for developing a broader international network in the future building on some of the great connections that have already been made. Examples of this emergent international collaboration includes the Derby Manager Neil Woodhead supporting Western Australian conversations and the growing links between Singapore and some of the UK programmes, particularly Swansea.

Besides a focus with existing members, the Network also plays the crucial role in supporting new areas wishing to adopt Local Area Coordination in England and Wales. It achieves this by collaborating with them in all aspects of their design, development and implementation through a defined piece of contracted work before that area eventually becomes a regular member themselves. This has proven to be a critical investment. As each new area joins, new learning from existing ones is passed along as leaders and Coordinators connect with each other across the Network. This strengthens the design process and creates more sustainable conditions for local growth through natural supportive relationships brokered through the Network – this is a clear example of how the principles of Local Area Coordination are themselves enshrined in the ethos of the Network. This virtuous circle of learning is then fed back into the wider Network as new areas reflect upon and share what has worked well and what hasn't in their local context. An example of this in the ongoing development of a shared learning and evaluation framework that also can adapt strategically to each local context.

This collective and collaborative leadership (at all levels) has meant that Local Area Coordination in England and Wales has grown in line with its core principles and design features. However, beyond that is has achieved its aspiration to become the central repository for Local Area Coordination knowledge and a unique and powerful collective of change-makers in England and Wales. The future is exciting for the Network, especially as the prospect of new international collaborations develop with potential for a more defined global movement to be shaped and led by constituent organisations.

126

7.2 International Initiative for Disability Leadership

by Eddie Bartnik

The International Initiative for Disability Leadership (IIDL) is an international membership organisation which focuses on collective and inclusive leadership development and the rapid dissemination of policy, research, resources and innovative practice across the eight member countries Australia, New Zealand, England, Scotland, Ireland, Sweden, Canada and the Unites States. Countries join as members and leaders can then participate for free and pay only for their travel. The signature activity of IIDL is an international leadership exchange and network meeting every 18-24 months, rotating between member countries and shared with their umbrella network the International Initiative for Mental Health Leadership (IIMHL).

As part of the 2018 International Leadership Exchange and Network Meeting held in Sweden, three organisations came together to host a two-day Local Area Coordination Leadership Exchange in Thurrock, England:

- **Local Area Coordination Network CIC** – the not-for-profit organisation supporting the design, implementation and long-term sustainability of Local Area Coordination in England and Wales
- **Inclusive Neighbourhoods Ltd** – led by Ralph Broad who founded the Local Area Coordination Network through supporting the early developments in England and Wales and now works elsewhere across Europe and internationally supporting Local Area Coordination and associated developments
- **Thurrock Council** – one of the first Councils in England to develop Local Area Coordination, now having sustained and grown the programme as an integral part of their wider asset-based approach in how health & social care work with local people, communities and organisations

127

They were joined by 10 international visitors from Australia, Canada and New Zealand, 2 colleagues from other Local Area Coordination programmes in Swansea and the Isle of Wight, 20 Community members, and workers from across Thurrock who have direct experience of Local Area Coordination, the Chief Social Worker for Adults (England) and Chair of TLAP (Think Local Act Personal) in England.

The Exchange focused on sharing the evidence, learning and real experiences of people delivering, experiencing or working with Local Area Coordination. The work in England and Wales was the starting point but international experiences and evidence were shared through the Exchange.

The presentations, resources and core information shared through the exchange can be found online at the Local Area Coordination Network.

The key messages from the Exchange were shared at the International Initiative for Disability Leadership Network meeting in Sweden:

- Local Area Coordination has a sound and growing international evidence base
- We are all on the same reform journey with same challenges
- Power of relationships
- The focus on a good life, a positive vision, strengths
- Importance of shifting power from systems to citizens
- Integrity and authenticity – person by person, family by family, place by place
- Leadership – 'How to develop tomorrow's leaders?'
- Imagine if... possibilities, possibilities, possibilities

The International Initiative for Disability Leadership continues to provide a helpful vehicle for international collaboration amongst the Local Area Coordination international connections. For example, recent 2020 webinars hosted by Think Local Act Personal (TLAP) and IIDL featuring Australia's National Disability Insurance Scheme (NDIS) have also highlighted the role of Local Area Coordination as a fundamental part of this world-first transformative Scheme. The next International Leadership Exchange is in Christchurch 2022 and provides another opportunity for an international Local Area Coordination Leadership exchange hosted either in Australia or New Zealand.

On a practical level, IIDL provides a platform for rapid sharing of new information as well as a way of building smaller networks and collaborations, as featured in the two examples below. Baptcare in Tasmania, Australia have commenced a research project on Supported Decision Making with Dr Michael Kendrick and a group of expert people with lived experience, academics, policy makers and practitioners. The project is seeking to understand what people who appoint a nominee, or who are a nominee, understand about the role of a nominee and how it helps them to make decisions and lead a life with choice and control. As part of the project, Baptcare is also collating websites, research and information available to the wider community so as to create a library of resources.

Catherine Viney from Baptcare leads their work on Local Area Coordination and writes:

"This work came about as a direct result of Baptcare's connection with IIDL, firstly in our participation in conversations about Local Area Coordination in 2018 in the Thurrock UK exchange, and then last year in Washington DC where one of our leaders, Emily Daniels, was challenged and inspired by the work of those facilitating the IIDL Leadership Exchange on Supported Decision Making. The value of IIDL for us at Baptcare is in using the expertise and enthusiasm of leading thinkers internationally to support us to improve our practice in the local communities that we work in."

The second example was a follow up event that considered reflections on Local Area Coordination when at its best in Western Australia, including the role of family leadership. The impetus for this informal network event came from the May 2018 Local Area Coordination Leadership Exchange held in Thurrock, London as part of the International Initiative for Disability Leadership (IIDL). Eddie Bartnik and Catherine Viney were part of that event and were keen to set up a broad international Local Area Coordination network through IIDL. Both Baptcare and the West Australian Department of Communities were reviewing international best practice for Local Area Coordination and this event was part of that discovery process.

The gathering was held in Perth on the 24th of June 2018 with a group of leaders with deep experience of Local Area Coordination since the 1990s in Western Australia, and some keen people looking to learn from the long-term experience of when 'Local Area Coordination was at its best' in the original location in WA. The format of the evening was informal and each participant was invited to share stories and examples which illustrated Local Area Coordination at its best in WA; not to dwell on how or why circumstances had changed or the current situation, but rather to elicit some depth of information through collective reflection that would add value to the written literature. Participants were encouraged to focus on those examples that generated the most passion or depth of meaning for themselves.

The event report (Bartnik, 2018) included a summary of fundamental 'good' elements of early Local Area Coordination practice contributing to it being recognised as a highly innovative, effective and respected programme that benefited the lives of many Western Australians with disability, their families and carers, as well as the broader WA community.

In particular, the report highlighted a number of unique perspectives from the long-term example, that are not often captured in the literature on Local Area Coordination:

- **Partnerships with families and strong family leadership** - There was equality between Local Area Coordinators and families with families leading and respected for their natural authority. Local Area Coordinators recognised that it was critical to work with the whole family unit, rather than just the individual. Investment was made in families to build their leadership capacity and strengthen their voice by offering training opportunities and inviting them to present at Disability Services Commission planning days. Local Area Coordination was about building individual and family capacity. A family member once stated to a consultative group that, "My Local Area coordinator teaches me how to catch fish as opposed to catching the fish for me."
- **Values, skills and the fundamental importance of training or annual forums** - The training was not only attended by Local Area Coordinators, but also by people with disability, their families and carers, government and community agencies, in order to create a learning exchange and to ensure the training remained relevant and based on lived experiences. Families learning in these settings subsequently realised higher expectations for their family member with a disability. This is particularly relevant for envisioning and has been considered by some of the participants as inspirational and life changing.
- **Leadership that was collective, connected and consistent** - Consistency of leadership was critical in maintaining the original intent of Local Area Coordination. Through consistent leadership, the values that underpinned Local Area Coordination, and the community development role played by Local Area Coordinators, were upheld. It also meant that the programme was able to exist in its most innovative and creative form, rather than be systemised, for a long time. Local Area Coordination was the face of the Disability Services Commission in the community, families could see allies in Local Area Coordination right up the ladder.

129

7.3 Swansea's leadership group

by Councillor Mark Child

Once Senior Leadership, that is the political leadership and the top Corporate Director, decided that we had to address demand, we had to prevent demand, and the way we were going to do it was with Local Area Co-ordination, then we never called it a trial or a pilot, it was always just the start. This demonstrated a commitment and an ambition.

Within the Council the argument about demographics was obvious, we all knew austerity was going to affect budgets. We wanted to remain being Swansea Council, with the multitude of statutory and non-statutory functions actively undertaken, and not morph into Swansea Social Services Board. It was in their interests to support prevention, and those on the strategic front line were saying Local Area Coordination was the tool.

We knew Local Area Coordinators had to embed themselves into communities, but also earn the respect of service providers in those communities, the Police, the GPs, the community mental health teams, the Housing providers, the 3rd sector etc. It was also clear that prevention of need, or as we have learnt to say, enabling someone to have a good life, will clearly have benefits across all service sectors, despite it being unquantifiable in each person's life. We simply transposed the internal argument to an external one.

We went out selling Local Area Coordination, almost literally going door to door asking people to join and contribute. So, through sharing the same prevention agenda, and being a beneficiary of Local Area Coordination, a Leadership group of interested parties was set up to learn from and guide the expansion and deepening of Local Area Coordination in Swansea.

We had to resist internal pressures and ways of working; to have genuinely committed long term partners, they had to have a say. This also had implications for where the Local Area Coordinators should work, how they were to be employed, who they were accountable to. This process brought many individuals and organisations on board. The desire to improve peoples lives and prevent need for service intervention were the pre-requisites for participation in the Group, not any resource commitment.

We have found that most organisations are more dynamic than the Council, so that occasionally they are stepping ahead, driving Local Area Coordination. This has rubbed off on the council, forcing changes. Where previously an individual's assessed need might have demonstrated a gap in the service that needed to be filled, now the individual didn't need a service, so the gap disappeared.

We have had participation in the Leadership Group from Coastal, Pobl and Family local Registered Social Landlords (RSLs), Swansea Council for Voluntary Service, Citizens Advice, South Wales Police, Mid and West Wales Fire service, Swansea Bay Health Board, Swansea University, along with Swansea Council Social Services and its Poverty & Prevention section too. With a partnership leading Local Area Coordination, it also gets a head start wherever it expands to, with professionals and organisations there having already bought in to the idea and experienced it in practice. Within the council, having other local organisations come on board, both with the concept, the practicalities of implementing it, and sometimes even paying, has helped silence the cynics and answer the critics.

130

We want to continue growing in ownership, in embedding Local Area Coordination in Swansea. Currently Local Area Coordination is ostensibly run by the council, but I would like to see it embedded in a joint structure; in Wales this would be the Public Service Board or the Regional Partnership Board. This would have pooled budget and a shared ownership and would bring in others too.

It has always been in our minds to involve local corporate responsibility, the University has been pushing this idea, but we couldn't think of a way in, there were no existing shared structures and relationships. However, through the pandemic, businesses of all sizes have contributed help to local communities, through donations of money, or materials, or employees time, or facilities, and we are collecting all their names, to say thank you and then to see if we can translate this into a longer-term link with their communities via Local Area Coordination.

131

7.4 A new social contract between citizen & state

by Professor Donna Hall, CBE

I started my local government career in Leeds City Council in the 1980s in the middle of a recession and have spent most of the time between then and now working on local economic regeneration projects in the north of England and eventually becoming a chief executive in three councils, most recently Wigan Council where we developed a new social contract with citizens, *The Wigan Deal*.

What really motivated me on a personal level was a growing sense of disappointment and frustration that regeneration initiatives I had worked on, whether physical or community based, didn't stick. They didn't really make a long-lasting difference. After we had spent £25 million, the place still had the same if not worse health indicators, people still had low paid or no employment and they tended to die earlier than their wealthier neighbours outside of the regeneration zone. I wanted to do something when I became a chief executive that would make a genuine and lasting difference to people, to families, to communities, to neighbourhoods.

What we needed was a new long term, all embracing social contract with residents; to be confident enough to have different conversations with each other about how we could work better together and grow the social scaffolding in a place. Stop well-meaning but siloed professionals all separately interacting with people, trying to prescribe for them, trying to 'fix' them without knowing them or understanding the reality of their lives.

The Wigan Deal was a response initially to austerity as Wigan was the third worst cut council back in 2011 when it began. We had a burning platform having to save £160 million from our revenue budgets. We knew we needed to think completely differently about the role of public services working together in a place if we were to survive and protect our residents from the worst aspects of austerity and welfare reform.

We invested £12 million in grassroots community projects designed to promote good physical and mental health and to grow the social infrastructure. We had £160 million to save but what we had was our people and many more assets that we could build on, so we focused on these assets in our communities, small groups of neighbours, a run-down community centre, a passionate GP, a teacher who had ambition for her children's and their families and we started to support residents to their own social movement.

We brought together multidisciplinary teams across social care, police, housing, NHS etc. to work together in integrated place-based teams, sharing data and supporting people to lead their best lives rather than interacting with them separately in an expensive and disjointed way without seeing the human being and treating them as a unit of need in a revolving door of services. We allowed the frontline workers in these teams to try new things and to innovate, to be radical innovators only doing things that actually helped the person or the family rather than continuing to assess and refer them without really listening to them or helping them in any meaningful way.

We are very lucky to have the Local Area Coordination Network supporting a wide range of councils, their partners and local community organisations. It is essential that we learn from each other and build on the brilliant examples that we can see springing up in pockets across the UK. If we are to support a whole system social movement, we need to work together to embed Local Area Coordination across public services.

132

Anthropology was at the heart of the change and used to help us develop tools and techniques to change the way we listened as an organisation to our own staff and more importantly to our communities. It was much more than social prescribing, which is still a power relationship that is based on the prescriber holding the power and the passive recipient of services on the receiving end. This was a new relationship, a new permanent social contract and an investment in prevention, wellbeing, resilience and confidence.

If we are to deliver real and lasting change, we need to work differently with communities over the long term, to rebuild trust and respect and to ensure we wrap supports and services around them through Local Area Coordination, not keep expecting them to navigate the current complexity. We need to build on the strengths that exist already within a person, a family, a street, a community and do all we can to build up these strengths rather than focus on the deficit-based models beloved of public services historically. It really works and unleashes a positive passion and energy from staff and neighbours - an energy that we desperately need in current times.

133

8. Call to action

During the writing of this book, we have engaged many of our long-term leaders and collaborators in sharing their experiences and hopes for Local Area Coordination in the currently fast changing pandemic and digital world. There is a strong commitment and interest to accelerate reforms rather than let things slip back to old models and traditional systems. It is a critical time to be clear about the sort of future we want for our citizens, local communities and society overall.

Local Area Coordination has more than 30 years of growing and uninterrupted learning and evidence across population groups, settings and contexts. The research evidence clearly shows that when implemented with fidelity, we can expect strong and consistent value for money outcomes at the levels of individual and family, local community and overall services system, with strong alignment to national and local policy and strategic priorities. We reassert our bold vision for Local Area Coordination in light of a rapidly changing world and call all potential collaborators to action.

134

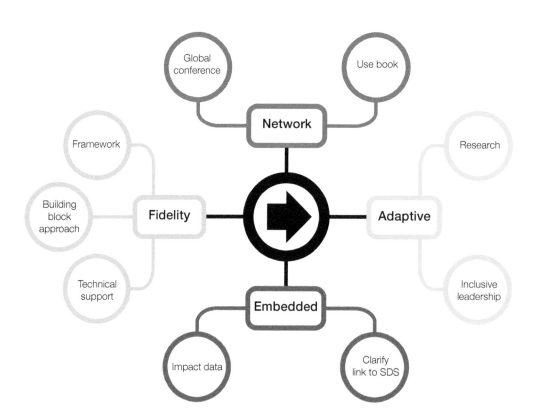

FIGURE 20. Strategic Actions Areas to bring Local Area Coordination to Full International Potential

Our 2026 vision is that we ensure a high level of fidelity, quality and sustainability of all current Local Area Coordination sites and simultaneously also continue to grow Local Area Coordination to new settings and populations and scale up to complete geographical coverage in those locations.

There are four key strategic directions and nine action areas in our forward 5-year plan to bring this vision to reality and we need leaders and collaborators at every level of the social care and health system and in the community. As Al Etmanski describes, we need disruptive innovators, bridging innovators and receptive innovators through a movement of collective and inclusive leadership.

1. A building blocks approach to ensure fidelity

One of our most powerful learnings has been that we need to be crystal clear about fidelity – in particular, the connected role of the Local Area Coordinator and the direct placement in and strong connection of the role to community. Fidelity is about understanding, delivering and improving 'what works', the key conditions for sustainable individual, family and community led outcomes and systems change. Where some countries and localities have 'cherry picked' or split up the various components of the Local Area Coordinator role, the results have also been proportionally diminished.

There are three key actions proposed. **First**, to use the 'Building blocks' approach outlined in Chapter 3 through the further development and then use of self-assessment and training resources which more clearly and directly state what Local Area Coordination is and is not. A commitment to ongoing learning and development is essential. **Second**, is the regular updating and refreshing of the Local Area Coordination Framework. This process would be enhanced through an international collaborative network and the shared commitment to a common Framework and operating approach, whilst acknowledging the importance of local context and strategic positioning. This relates to preserving the core values and principles of Local Area Coordination, whilst at the same time stimulating change and progress. **Third**, to expand the base of credible and skilled technical support to address all fidelity criteria so that quality and sustainability are in built rather than added on considerations.

135

2. An International learning network of all Local Area Coordination sites

We have a wonderful foundation to build from which is the partnership which has created this current publication, namely the England and Wales Local Area Coordination Network hosted by Community Catalysts CIC, Inclusive Neighbourhoods Ltd and Tamar Consultancy Pty Ltd. The Centre for Welfare Reform is also a significant source of valuable information, resources, learning and connections, including the Citizen Network.

A fundamental building block of Local Area Coordination is 'Nationally shared values and Framework, regular connections through a network with international best practice connections'.

A practical example of the power of such connection and collaboration is the long-term evidence from Western Australia with people with disabilities which inspired and supported the original work in England and Wales alongside a broader range of health and social care populations beyond disability. The cycle continued where the evidence from England and Wales then inspired the recent first Australian project in Western Australia beyond disability and so this high degree of reciprocity and learning continues.

Strong efforts are being made currently to strengthen the connection of all Local Area Coordinators internationally. These efforts include:

- The 2020 England and Wales Local Area Coordination Network Annual Gathering which was progressively opened up to collaborators from a range of international sites.
- The production of this international publication with a wide range of contributing authors will also serve to build bridges between our various sites internationally and inspire potential collaborators to take action.
- A further example is the growing partnership with the International Initiative for Disability Leadership which provides an excellent opportunity for hosted Leadership Exchanges that build on the Thurrock 2018 Local Area Coordination Exchange. Following the next International Exchange and Network meeting to be held in Christchurch, New Zealand in 2022, the Exchange returns to the Netherlands in 2024 which would provide an ideal opportunity for another international hosted event in the United Kingdom.

There are two key actions proposed. **First,** to use this new book as a means to re-connect with all Local Area Coordination sites across the world and invite them into our collective effort. **Second,** to work in partnership to host an annual international event that is open to all Local Area Coordination sites across the world.

3. Embed Local Area Coordination into system reforms

This relates to what we call 'Connecting the dots of reform and system transformation' and positioning Local Area Coordination strategically and effectively as part of reforms and strategic linkages in each jurisdiction. Local Area Coordination can serve as a key catalyst for whole human services system transformation.

A good example of this comes from the very first Local Area Coordination site in Western Australia and the simultaneous development of Local Area Coordination with direct consumer funding or what is now called personal budgets. The move to personalised and localised support is substantially strengthened when people have a greater degree of control of any supports or services they might require. In essence, and as set out in the Local Area Coordination principles, it is a matter of the best balance between informal, community and mainstream supports and then any paid services that may be required to complement rather than replace these informal supports and mainstream services.

This rebalancing of the Local Area Coordinator role in some settings requires stronger partnerships between Local Area Coordination and personal budgets in the UK for example and in Australia a refocus on the informal, community and mainstream aspects of the role with less focus on the personal budgets.

A further aspect of this strategic positioning is the development of relationships and cross sector leadership which enables creative resourcing involving a combination of recycled and new resources as well as pooled funding from different silos.

There are two key actions proposed. **First,** to strengthen impact data to inform system reform, as it has been clearly demonstrated that through time and systematic application, Local Area Coordination has a transformative effect in the wider service system beyond

136

those changes that were needed in the first place to establish. This 'virtuous circle' of improvement marks a discrete step in our learning about the wider impact of Local Area Coordination since the publication of the last paper in 2015. **Second**, to resolve the right relationship between Local Area Coordination and the parallel work on personal budgets and self-directed support. Getting crystal clear on this relationship will strengthen both fidelity and quality of Local Area Coordination practice as well as sustainability and bringing to full scale and coverage in each location. An effective relationship between Local Area Coordination and personal budgets will also contribute to better access to and more effective use of personal budgets. We also know that the lives of people are enhanced when they can determine their preferred supports and services, to the extent that they desire.

4. Learn, adapt and thrive

An ongoing commitment to review, reflect and improve all aspects of Local Area Coordination, from design and practice to leadership is required to continue to support the evolution, relevance and impact of Local Area Coordination alongside local people and communities and to stimulate change within the service system. This building block has been described earlier as "An open culture characterised by participation, feedback, reviews and evaluations and independent monitoring." Where sites have been able to scale to full coverage, these have all been punctuated by regular independent evaluations and research which continue to demonstrate the outcomes and value for money of the Local Area Coordination approach.

These evaluations also serve to bring implementation back to the core principles and design features, as all service systems have a tendency to draw innovative initiatives back to more traditional practice.

There are two key actions proposed. **First**, to require regular independent evaluations as a core condition of demonstrating fidelity and quality and to grow the network of universities and independent evaluators. **Second**, a commitment to collective and inclusive leadership, both within and across sectors, with a growing focus on inequalities and people who services find it hard to support.

There is a substantial body of work ahead but also a wonderful opportunity. We have had 30 years of conventional wisdom saying 'this will never work' or 'we are already doing that'. We also now have 30 years of strong and growing evidence that Local Area Coordination does work effectively across settings and population groups, and that where people have the courage to stick with the evidence and not compromise, this is what ultimately leads to the marked improvements in outcomes for the people and communities we support, 'one good life at a time'.

We invite you to join us on this journey and join our international Local Area Coordination community.

137

AFTERWORD

by Dr Michael J. Kendrick

If one were to choose a title for an insurgent and inspired attempt to positively transform the lives of persons with disabilities or mental health needs, it is quite unlikely that the seemingly highly bureaucratic sounding term 'Local Area Coordination' would initially come to mind. Yet, in my experience with Local Area Coordination, what I witnessed was a systematic and self-consciously deliberative strategic effort to do just that, to make it possible for people to have genuinely good lives, irrespective of the specific disabilities and impairments they lived with. To say that this effort was systematic in nature would be an understatement, as it was well led at many levels and in many dimensions of people's lives by carefully selected and passionately committed Local Area Coordinators. The reference to the 'local areas' that the Local Area Coordination programme intentionally and self-consciously partnered with were the many people, groups, resources, life opportunities and potential allies that constitute local communities. The vision being that Local Area Coordinators, in cooperation with the person, their families, personal networks and more broadly with diverse elements the community at large, provided a rich array of potential pathways to personally fulfilling lives.

The Local Area Coordination strategy and ethos unfolded through the presence and engagement of many people who could best be described as de facto 'community partners' with the Local Area Coordination strategy, whether they were particularly mindful of this role or not. This included employers, neighbours, teachers, club members, housemates in some instances, church members, support circle members and so on. Of course, this was a deliberate effect of the Local Area Coordination strategy of enabling people with disabilities or other needs to ultimately enjoy good lives of their own making as fully as possible within the wealth of potential life opportunities available in many diverse communities. Subsequently, I was to see the same pattern emerge in other states and countries. What was being created, nurtured and evolved was, in essence, thousands of different versions of 'the good life', one person at a time. Yes, it was always local and involved 'coordination' with all manner of people. However, what made it notable was all of what gradually changed for the better in people's lives.

The founding of Local Area Coordination was in the state of Western Australia. It occurred there because of the visionary leadership of the mix of state officials and leaders within that system who created, evolved, implemented, financed, defended, problem solved, found state financing for and ultimately nurtured and evolved the local area coordination effort, both within the context of state government and the community at large. At all levels, the Local Area Coordination programme was funded and operated as a regular component of state government and consequently had to competently and skilfully adhere to the many requirements of the state bureaucratic systems, policies, budgets and politics. Part of that skilful adherence involved the process of 'bureaucratic shielding' of as much of the local area programme 'on the ground' from the normal politics, agendas and financial concerns of any state government. This occurred simultaneously with finding often novel ways to creatively translate needs at the personal and community level into strategies that could succeed within the often arcane and potentially conflictual agendas common to most government departments, political parties and outside constituencies.

Another central term that comes to mind that characterised the Local Area Coordination programme in multiple jurisdictions overall was 'visionary'. The Local Area Coordination leaders internationally have been intensely interested in what was considered 'leading edge' emergent best and were quite consciously investing in bringing the ideas and people behind these to their jurisdictions. In the process 'seeding' their adoption and nurture as part of the moral, ideological and practice aspects of the vision that guided their sense of what the 'good life' could potentially be for people with disabilities. Over the years that included now recognised 'best practice' elements such as supported employment, social role valorisation, social inclusion, person centred practice and lifestyles, empowerment, individualised funding, 'home of one's own', independent advocacy, safeguards and vulnerability, 'right relationship', micro-enterprises, service user and family governed service models, community membership, innovation, developmental growth, rights, adaptive technology, microboards, supported decision making, optimal individual service design, leadership development and self-direction to name just a few. Today, many of these practices have become mainstream. However, what is striking is how often the Local Area Coordination programmes adopted their use at a very early stage in the innovation adoption curve which reflects the early uptake of leading-edge innovations. Taken together, these and other influences provided a rich, mutually reinforcing and cross-fertilising supply of insight and inspiration to challenge Local Area Coordination to keep evolving in its sense of the what the true potentials of the 'good life' could become real for greater number if sufficient values based leadership was sustained.

139

The very fact that Local Area Coordination has both been transported into quite different governmental systems and has continued to innovate and evolve, is a striking endorsement of its potential adaptive capacities and the ultimate worth of its vision for the people it is attempting to support. Perhaps even more important is that it has been attractive to the leaders in those systems who are looking for trustworthy strategies that could reliably generate good quality of life outcomes, even in environments and communities that are extremely diverse, strained and limited by their own hindrances. A key aspect of Local Area Coordination is that it cannot work to realise its many potential benefits without the presence of such leaders that both see its promise and personally have the initiative, adaptive leadership skills and abilities to get real results irrespective of the challenges involved. Local Area Coordination could not optimise its potential beneficial outcomes without the quality of these leaders.

Going forward it would be useful for those involved to reflect upon the optimal character of the relationship between engaged leaders and the optimisation of the complex, but positive programmatic potentials inherent in Local Area Coordination practice. One lesson that comes from sustained Local Area Coordination experience is that it has consciously engaged a diverse mix of leaders both within and outside of itself in variations of alliances of shared purpose and values at both a local community level, but also more broadly including numerous international linkages and collaborations.

Notably, some of those leaders were not part of the bureaucratic systems that hosted Local Area Coordination, but rather were external allies acting in concert with leaders in formal roles within the Local Area Coordination bureaucratic system. If you like, there would be much value to be gained from appraising the value and contribution of these forms of 'collective' rather than solely 'individual' leadership and its relationship to ultimate outcomes. Further, the Local Area Coordination experience is very instructive in terms of the intentional creation of an overall ecology of multi-level partnerships and alliances in support of important values and outcomes. Not an easy challenge to be sure, but it is much easier knowing what has already been accomplished, not only in a few, but now many jurisdictions.

What has been said here has been from the vantage point of looking back at what has already transpired. Of course, if the Local Area Coordination approach is to have a future, its current leaders and supporters must necessarily look beyond what has already been accomplished to the question of what might be the other potential ways that the Local Area Coordination approach could or should evolve further. This concern should not be framed solely in terms of what might conceivably benefit Local Area Coordination and the people and communities it currently supports (for example, increasing the fidelity of implementation in some current sites), but rather what might be optimal or 'best practice' given the diverse needs of people in coming decades. That may include people whose needs differ from the growing number of groups already supported to perhaps people who have engaged in crime or people from other cultural groups at risk of mistreatment, marginalisation or neglect. This could include groups that are currently or historically unassimilated and at the margins of society, such as is common with indigenous peoples or other historically socially excluded groups.

What might be provoked by such speculations is what has been learned thus far from the Local Area Coordination journey that could conceivably benefit persons or groups it has not yet engaged with, even if it means evolving new variants in terms of overall Local Area Coordination practice. It would not be surprising in such instances that Local Area Coordination may be currently unready for such challenges, given how it presently is constituted. Nonetheless, being unready at one point in time does not necessarily mean that it cannot gradually adapt such that it builds the missing capacities it will need. These could include linguistic and cultural capacities, new methods of support and community mobilisation to meet needs, increased consciousness and awareness of the spiritual and psychological ethos of a socially marginalised group, competence with ethical partnering in new ways and so on.

There is wisdom in not taking on challenges that one is unready for, but there is also the wisdom of knowing that with time such readiness can be cultivated. Thus, creating the opportunity to eventually address distinct human needs and challenges that are currently not being well met. There is no shortage of people and groups who are suffering and oppressed, whose lives might look very different in coming years if they were to have available to them the precisely 'right' kinds of support that would help them thrive. This would include new people and places as well as existing Local Area Coordination sites where current practice can be improved and lifted to optimal performance.

It may seem strange to end an 'afterword' with a speculative look forward. However, it does reinforce the assumption that Local Area Coordination has a future it must consider, not merely a past to chronicle. That has always been true for Local Area Coordination and it explains its ongoing evolution. Hopefully, that ongoing evolution will also be captured in further writings or books on Local Area Coordination in coming years.

140

BIBLIOGRAPHY

Bartnik E (2018) *Reflections on Local Area Coordination when at its best in Western Australia*. Available from: http://inclusiveneighbourhoods.co.uk/reflections-on-local-area-coordination-when-at-its-best-in-western-australia/

Bartnik E (2007) *Local Area Coordination in the Australian Capital Territory: External Evaluation Summary Report*. Canberra: Australian Capital Territory. Available from: http://inclusiveneighbourhoods.co.uk/lac-in-ausct/

Bartnik E & Chalmers R (2007) *It's about more than the money: Local Area Coordination Supporting People with Disabilities* in S Hunter & P Ritchie (eds) *Co-Production and Personalisation in Social Care: Changing relationships in the provision of social care*. London: Jessica Kingsley

Bartnik E & Psaila-Savona S (2003) *Value for money. Paper for the Local Area Coordination Review Steering Committee*. Western Australia. Available from: http://inclusiveneighbourhoods.co.uk/review-of-the-lac-w-aus/

Broad R (2012) *Local Area Coordination - From Service Users to Citizens*. Sheffield: Centre for Welfare Reform. Available from: http://inclusiveneighbourhoods.co.uk/from-service-users-to-citizens/

Broad R (2015) *People, Places, Possibilities*. Sheffield: Centre for Welfare Reform. Available from: http://inclusiveneighbourhoods.co.uk/people-places-possibilities/

Centre for Liveable Cities (2019) *Age Friendly Cities - Lessons from Seoul and Singapore*. Singapore: Centre for Liveable Cities.

Chadbourne R (2003) *A review of research on Local Area Coordination in Western Australia. Consultant's report to the Local Area Coordination Steering Committee*. Perth: Edith Cowan University.

Chenoweth L & Stehlik D (2002) *Building the Capacity of Individuals, Families and Communities: Evaluation of the Local Area Coordination Pilot Programme*. Brisbane: QLD: Disability Services Queensland. Available from: http://inclusiveneighbourhoods.co.uk/wp-content/uploads/2020/11/2002-QLD-Building-the-capacity-of-individuals-families-and-communities.pdf

Collins J C & Porras J I (2005) *Built to last: Successful habits of visionary companies*. New York: Random House.

Darnton P, Slden J, Liles A, Sibley A, Anstee S, Brooks C & Benson T (2018) *Independent Evaluation of Local Area Coordination on the Isle of Wight*. Wessex: AHSN. Available from: https://bit.ly/2Gfxois [Accessed 06/02/2021]

Care Act (2014) United Kingdom

Derby City Council (2020) *Local Area Coordination in Derby; Evaluation report 2018-20*. Publication Pending

Design Singapore Council (2020) *Building a Healthcare Hub in the North*. Available from: https://www.designsingapore.org/stories/building-a-healthcare-hub-in-the-north.html [Accessed 06/02/2021]

Elby D (2015) *Rx: The Quiet Revolution*. Available from: https://www.pbs.org/video/wttw-featured-rx-quiet-revolution/ [Accessed 06/02/2021]

Etmanski A (2015) Impact: Six patterns to spread your social innovation. Orwell Cove.

Gamsu M & Rippon S (2019) *Making Haringey a Better Place... where everyone can thrive*. Available at: https://lacnetwork.org/wp-content/uploads/2019/06/June-2019-Haringey-formative-evaluation.pdf

Government of Western Australia (2003) *Review of the Local Area Coordination Program Western Australia*. Available from: http://inclusiveneighbourhoods.co.uk/review-of-the-lac-w-aus/

iF World Design Guide (2017) *iF Social Impact Prize 2017*. Available from: https://ifworlddesignguide.com/entry/238094-share-a-pot [Accessed 06/02/2021]

Jones D (2020) *Circling the Square: Cwmbwrla, Coronavirus and Community*. Independently Published.

141

Kendrick M (1997) *Leadership and service quality.* International Social Role Valorisation Journal, 2, 2, Autumn, pp. 62-68

Kingfishers Ltd (2015) *The Social Value of Local Area Coordination in Thurrock. A Forecast Social Return on Investment Analysis for Adult Social Care, Thurrock.* Available from: http://inclusiveneighbourhoods. co.uk/social-value-of-local-area-coordination-in-thurrock/

Kingfishers Ltd (2016) *Social Value of Local Area Coordination in Derby.* Available from: https:// www.thinklocalactpersonal.org.uk/_assets/Resources/BCC/Assured-SROI-Report-for-Local-Area-Coordination-in-Derby-March-2016.pdf

Lunt N & Bainbridge L (2019) *Local Area Coordination Summative Evaluation.* York: University of York. Available from: https://lacnetwork.org/wp-content/uploads/2019/04/190415-Local-Area-Coordination-Summative-Report-15_-4_19FINAL.pdf

Mason J, Oatley C, Harris K & Ryan L (2021) *How and why does Local Area Coordination work for people in Different Contexts?* Methodological Innovations, Vol. 14 Issue: 1, pp. 1-12 doi:10.1177/2059799120985381

M E L Research (2016) *Leicestershire Local Area Coordination Evaluation.* Available from: https://bit.ly/2VZFfIT [Accessed 06/02/2021]

Michael J (2019) *Independent Review of the Isle of Man Health and Social Care System.* Available from: https://www.gov.im/media/1365879/independent-health-and-social-care-review-final-report.pdf

Ministry of Health Singapore (2019) *Healthier Together – Empowering Singaporeans to care for ourselves and one another.* Available from: https://www.moh.gov.sg/docs/librariesprovider5/default-document-library/cos-booklet-design-draft-6-mar-1000hrs33dcd84cb634436ca4731b01926c9598.pdf

Mollidor C, Bierman R, Goujon C, Zanobetti L & Akhurst E (2020) *Evaluation of the Derby Local Area Coordination Approach.* Department for Education. Available from: https://assets.publishing. service.gov.uk/government/uploads/system/uploads/attachment_data/file/932029/Derby_Local_Area_Coordination.pdf

Moore M (2013) *Recognising public value.* Massachusetts: Harvard University Press.

National Disability Authority Ireland (2015) *Local Area Coordination Briefing Paper.* Available from: http://nda.ie/nda-files/NDA-Local-Area-Coordination-Briefing-paper-PDF-format-.pdf

NDIS (2021) *LAC partners in the Community.* Available from: https://www.ndis.gov.au/understanding/ what-ndis/whos-rolling-out-ndis/lac-partners-community [Accessed 01/03/2021]

NHS England (2014) *NHS Five Year Forward View.* Available from: https://www.england.nhs.uk/five-year-forward-view/ [Accessed 06/02/2021]

Oatley C (2016) *Local Area Coordination Formative Evaluation: Understanding the praxis and impact of the Local Area Coordination approach on the Isle of Wight.*
Available from: http://inclusiveneighbourhoods.co.uk/wp-content/uploads/2016/07/Local-Area-Coordination-Evaluation-Report-.pdf

Peter Fletcher Associates (2011) *Evaluation of Local Area Coordination in Middlesbrough.* Available from: https://www.centreforwelfarereform.org/uploads/attachment/318/evaluation-of-local-area-coordination.pdf

Pierce J C (2000) *The paradox of physicians and administrators in health care organizations.* Health Care Management Review, Vol.25 Iss: 1, pp.7-28

Productivity Commission (2011) *Disability Care and Support Report No. 54.* Canberra.

Productivity Commission (2017) *National Disability Insurance Scheme (NDIS) Costs Study Report Canberra.* Available from: https://www.pc.gov.au/inquiries/completed/ndis-costs/report/ndis-costs.pdf

Public Services Social Value Act (2012) United Kingdom

Roderick S, Davies G H, Daniels J & Gregory J (2016) *Local Community Initiatives in Western Bay.* Available at: https://bit.ly/2D9cEHc [Accessed 06/02/2021]

Roorda M, Nunns H, Goodwin D, Were L & Sullivan M (2014) *Evaluation of Local Area Coordination (New Zealand).* Wellington: Evalue Research.

142

Scottish Consortium for Learning Disability (2006) *Making Connections: Stories of Local Area Coordination in Scotland.* Available from: http://inclusiveneighbourhoods.co.uk/wp-content/uploads/2020/11/2006-Scotland-Stories-Making-Connections.pdf

Scottish Government (2008) *National Guidance on the Implementation of Local Area Coordination.* Available from: http://inclusiveneighbourhoods.co.uk/wp-content/uploads/2021/02/2008-National-Guidance-on-Implementation-of-LAC-.pdf

Scottish Executive (2000) *The same as you? A review of services for people with learning disabilities.* Edinburgh: The Stationary Office.

Social Services and Well-being (Wales) Act (2014) United Kingdom

Stalker K, Malloch M, Barry M & Watson J (2007) *Evaluation of the implementation of Local Area Coordination in Scotland.* Edinburgh: Scottish Executive.

Steering Committee for the Review of Commonwealth/State Service Provision (1998) *Implementing reforms in government services – Case study on Offering direct consumer funding and choice in WA disability services* (pp. 89-114). Canberra: AusInfo.

Tew J, Duggal S, Carr S, Ercolani M, Glasby J, Kinghorn P, Miller R, Newbigging K, Tanner D & Afentou N (2019) *Implementing the Care Act 2014: Building social resources to prevent, reduce or delay needs for care and support in adult social care in England. Final Report for the Department of Health and Social Care.* Available from: https://www.birmingham.ac.uk/schools/social-policy/departments/social-work-social-care/research/social-care-and-adult-well-being/care-act.aspx

Well-being of Future Generations (Wales) Act (2015) United Kingdom

Western Australia Department of Communities (2021) *Local Area Coordination Implementation Progress Evaluation.* Draft Unpublished.

Wong S F (2018) *A Case Study in Re-imagining Healthy Communities* in Chong KH & Cho M (Eds) *Creative Ageing Cities: Place Design with Older People in Asian Cities* (pp. 47- 60) doi:10.4324/9781315558684. London: Routledge.

143

APPENDICES

Below we have a series of images from Western Australia Department of Communities highlighting the key design conditions and practice that drive positive change at the individual, family, community and systems levels and examples illustrating this in action.

Firstly, we have 3 images that show an example of a logic model of the 'how and why' Local Area Coordination (Local Communities Coordination/LCC in Western Australia) design and practice drive positive outcomes alongside individuals and families, the communities in which they live and finally the wider service system.

We thank Western Australia Department of Communities and Social Ventures Australia (SVA) for giving permission to share these in the book.

Secondly, we have 2 info graphics from Western Australia Department of Communities. The first, shows the breadth and reach of Local Communities Coordination alongside people of different backgrounds – whole person, whole family, whole community. The second, shares a summary of outcomes, a powerful story of person led change from an individual who had an LCC alongside through difficult times and also feedback from both people who have accessed LCC and services who have worked in partnership with LCC.

144

We thank Western Australia Department of Communities for giving permission to share these in the book.

LCC Logic Model: Person level
Why and how does Your Toolkit work with people and what changes for them?

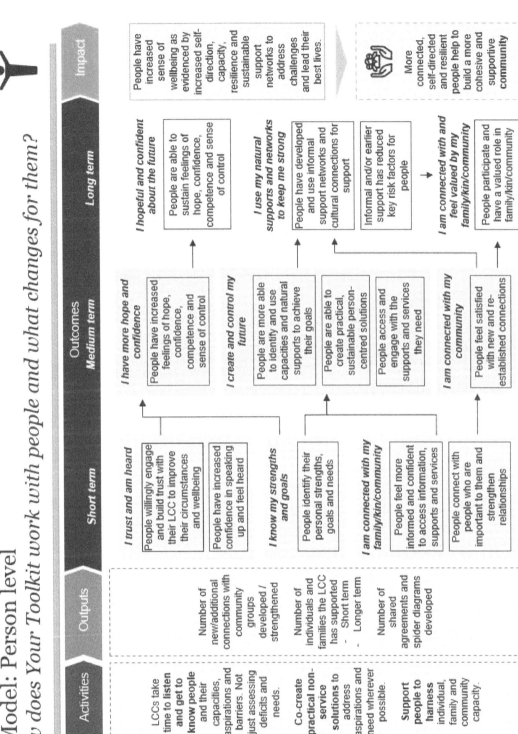

145

146

LCC Logic Model: Community level
Why and how do LCCs work with communities and what changes for them?

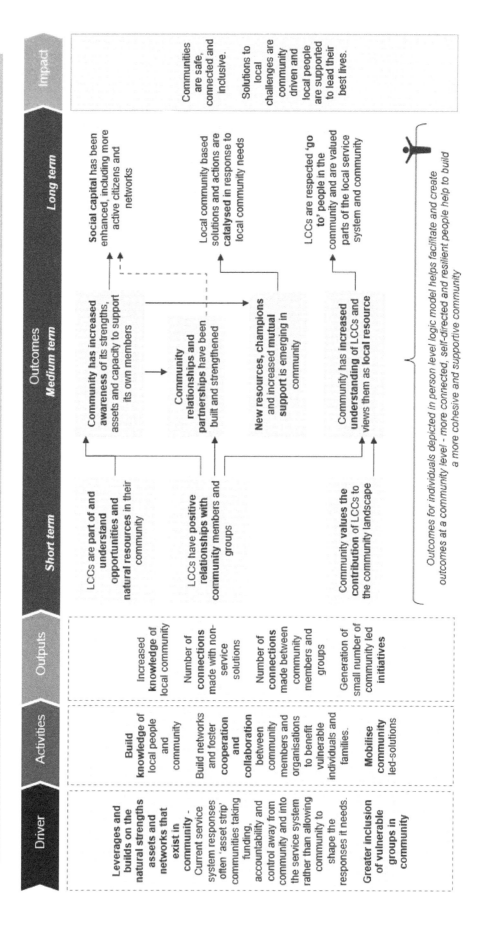

Driver	Activities	Outputs	Outcomes Short term	Outcomes Medium term	Outcomes Long term	Impact
Leverages and builds on the natural strengths assets and networks that exist in community - Current service system responses often 'asset strip' communities taking funding, accountability and control away from community and into the service system rather than allowing community to shape the responses it needs.

Greater inclusion of vulnerable groups in community | **Build knowledge of local people and community**

Build networks and foster cooperation and collaboration between community members and organisations to benefit vulnerable individuals and families.

Mobilise community led-solutions | Increased **knowledge** of local community

Number of **connections** made with non-service solutions

Number of **connections** made between community members and groups

Generation of small number of community led initiatives | LCCs are part of and understand **opportunities and natural resources** in their community

LCCs have positive **relationships** with community members and groups

Community values the contribution of LCCs to the community landscape | **Community has increased awareness** of its strengths, assets and capacity to support its own members

Community relationships and partnerships have been built and strengthened

New resources, champions and increased **mutual support** is emerging in community

Community has increased understanding of LCCs and views them as **local resource** | **Social capital has been enhanced**, including more active citizens and networks

Local community based solutions and actions are **catalysed** in response to local community needs

LCCs are respected **'go to'** people in the community and are valued parts of the local service system and community | Communities are safe, connected and inclusive.

Solutions to local challenges are community driven and local people are supported to lead their best lives. |

Outcomes for individuals depicted in person level logic model helps facilitate and create outcomes at a community level - more connected, self-directed and resilient people help to build a more cohesive and supportive community

LCC Logic Model: System level
Why and how do LCCs influence the system and what changes for the system?

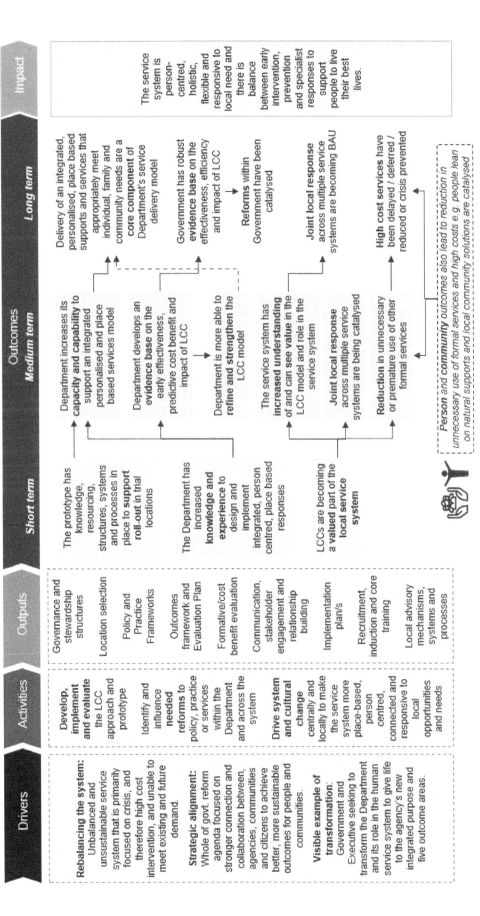

Drivers	Activities	Outputs	Outcomes — Short term	Outcomes — Medium term	Long term	Impact
Rebalancing the system: Unbalanced and unsustainable service system that is primarily focused on crisis, and therefore high cost intervention, and unable to meet existing and future demand.	**Develop, implement and evaluate** the LCC approach and prototype	Governance and stewardship structures	The prototype has knowledge, resourcing, structures, systems and processes in place to **support roll-out in trial locations**	Department increases its **capacity and capability** to support an integrated personalised and place based services model	Delivery of an integrated, personalised, place based supports and services that appropriately meet individual, family and community needs are a **core component** of Department's service delivery model	The service system is person-centred, holistic, flexible and responsive to local need and there is balance between early intervention, prevention and specialist responses to support people to live their best lives.
Strategic alignment: Whole of govt reform agenda focused on stronger connection and collaboration between, agencies, communities and citizens to achieve better, more sustainable outcomes for people and communities.	Identify and influence **needed reforms** to policy, practice or services within the Department and across the system	Location selection / Policy and Practice Frameworks	The Department has increased **knowledge and experience** to design and implement integrated, person centred, place based responses	Department develops an **evidence base** on the early effectiveness, predictive cost benefit and impact of LCC	Government has robust **evidence base** on the effectiveness, efficiency and impact of LCC	
Visible example of transformation: Government and Executive seeking to transform the Department and its role in the human service system to give life to the agency's new integrated purpose and five outcome areas.	**Drive system and cultural change** centrally and locally to make the service system more place-based, person centred, connected and responsive to local opportunities and needs	Outcomes framework and Evaluation Plan / Formative/cost benefit evaluation / Communication, stakeholder engagement and relationship building / Implementation plan/s / Recruitment, induction and core training / Local advisory mechanisms, systems and processes	LCCs are becoming a **valued part of the local service system**	Department is more able to **refine and strengthen the LCC model** / The service system has **increased understanding** of and can see value in the LCC model and role in the service system / **Joint local response** across multiple service systems are being catalysed / **Reduction in unnecessary** or premature use of other formal services	**Reforms within** Government have been catalysed / **Joint local response** across multiple service systems are becoming BAU / **High cost services** have been delayed / deferred / reduced or crisis prevented	

Person and community outcomes also lead to reduction in unnecessary use of formal services and high costs e.g. people lean on natural supports and local community solutions are catalysed

147

Local Communities Coordination Prototype
a whole person, whole family, whole community, whole system initiative

Local Communities Coordinators
have worked alongside

1,215
people*

670
Short Term

501
Long Term

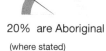

20% are Aboriginal
(where stated)

30% are people with a disability or carers or family of someone with a disability

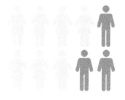

7 in 10 are women or girls

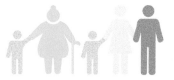

6 in 10 individuals supported long term live in a family group with dependent children
43% of those family groups include children aged 4 years or younger

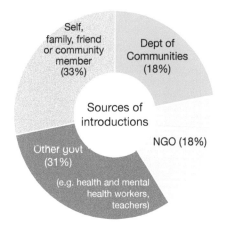

Sources of introductions

Self, family, friend or community member (33%)

Dept of Communities (18%)

NGO (18%)

Other govt (31%)
(e.g. health and mental health workers, teachers)

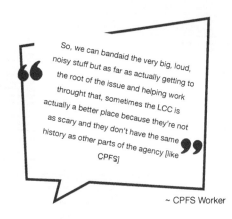

So, we can bandaid the very big, loud, noisy stuff but as far as actually getting to the root of the issue and helping work throught that, sometimes the LCC is actually a better place because they're not as scary and they don't have the same history as other parts of the agency [like CPFS]

~ CPFS Worker

Common challenges include

52% are experiencing housing stress or are homeless

47% have their daily life impacted by mental ill-health

18% have experienced family or domestic violence

62% of families present as overwhelmed

25% have had contact with Child Protection Services

Most people experience social isolation, which contributes to the other challenges they are facing

* as at 31 Dec 2020
** Nov 2020 data

POWER AND CONNECTION | APPENDICES

Local Communities Coordination Prototype
a whole person, whole family, whole community, whole system initiative

After explaining the role of a LCC and checking if he wanted to engage, the Dad replied ...

"Yes! I've never had access to this. I've been in crisis and ended up in psych units before but when they help you get over that it just ends. I just need help working out what to do because I'm ok at being a dad – I can feed them, put a roof over their head, but beyond that I'm not good at organising myself so that there's a routine or consistency and that's what they need."

We've got limited options to help people that either don't meet the child protection threshold or that we are no longer involved with ... we can refer them to the LCC and know that they are being supported

CPFS Team Leader

Through her own efforts Amy and her 7 children managed to escape a volatile and abusive relationship marked by violence and drug use. When she met with the LCC she was seeking support to rebuild family relationships, complete some training to get a job and improve her health. Her children are now safe and attending school. She wanted to be able to give her children "a life like other kids".

With the LCC's encouragement and support she enrolled them in vacation swimming classes and when it was time to go back to school sought some grant funding for school books and uniforms. Amy said her "kids were so excited they wanted to sleep in them". She has noticed a difference with her children actually wanting to go to school.

As more time passes Amy's confidence builds and she's feeling much more in control and able to make good decisions for herself and her children. Her positivity has filtered through to her children and they are finding home a far less stressful place to be. Amy is building connections into the community and is looking forward to doing some things for herself, like getting back into netball. She also feels ready to start looking for a job. A text message from Amy to the LCC reads, "thanks for sticking up for the strugglers"

Local Communities Coordination is making a difference:

- helping parents and carers who are overwhelmed and struggling to care for their loved ones
- supporting women and their children as they rebuild their lives after leaving violent relationships
- assisting people experiencing unstable housing or homelessness to access a range of housing options
- helping people living with a disability or mental health condition to find the supports and services they need, including NDIS
- helping people who are socially isolated to connect to family, friends, neighbours, peer or cultural groups that are important to them
- reducing the need for high cost interventions (e.g. out of home care, social housing, hospital admissions, etc.) as multiple underlying causes are addressed

149

"I'm thinking we have achieved getting me quite well re-integrated into society, and you have been so wonderful, supportive and effective in helping me do this."

~ Person accessing LCC

I'm a Paediatrician at the xx Child Development Service. I wanted to formally thank xxxx for the support he has recently provided to one of the vulnerable families I work with. He was able to address significant housing concerns for a single parent family with limited social support, recent family violence affecting the safety of the family in their previous accommodation and two children with very significant neurodevelopmental disabilities in a timely manner; and to assist this mother in progressing referrals and registrations for her children with the NDIS and therapy services. I recently reviewed this family again and they were in a much better position, with family stress significantly reduced and the mother and full time carer reporting significantly less stress and improved mood and optimism. It has also allowed their mother to continue to work. I would not have been able to achieve these outcomes in any other way and am extremely grateful to the professionalism and expertise of xxxx in this situation.

A REPORT FROM THE CENTRE FOR WELFARE REFORM

About the Authors

Eddie Bartnik has been continuously involved in Local Area Coordination from its inception in the late 1980s right through to the present. Further to his early role as state-wide Director of Local Area Coordination in Western Australia, he has been supporting Australian and international developments through his work as a Director of Tamar Consultancy Pty Ltd and his writings. Eddie has held a variety of senior state and national government positions across disability, mental health and community services, including being Western Australia's first Mental Health Commissioner and Strategic Advisor with the National Disability Insurance Scheme. He is currently International Lead for the International Initiative for Disability Leadership.

Ralph Broad is Director of Inclusive Neighbourhoods Ltd and led the development of Local Area Coordination in England and Wales. This built on the original ground-breaking developments in Western Australia, expanding Local Area Coordination to its current, inclusive "whole community, whole system" focus alongside people of all ages and backgrounds. He also established the England and Wales Local Area Coordination Network and authored the first two reports on Local Area Coordination in England and Wales. He has subsequently worked in partnership with leaders to support new Local Area Coordination developments in Western Australia, Singapore and now the Isle of Man, as part of contribution to health and social care reform. Prior to this, Ralph had a variety of senior leadership positions in organisations in England, Scotland and Western Australia.

150

About the Contributors

Al Etmanski is a community organiser and author. He's been a parent activist in the disability movement since his daughter Liz was born. Al is an Ashoka social entrepreneur fellow and member of John McKnight's Asset Based Community Development Institute. He has received the Order of Canada for his policy advocacy. His latest book is, The Power of Disability: 10 Lessons for Surviving, Thriving and Changing the World. He blogs at aletmanski.com.

Nick Sinclair leads on the development Local Area Coordination in England and Wales and convenes the Local Area Coordination Network. He previously worked for organisations alongside people facing homelessness and the issues surrounding it. He is the founding chair of Culture Connect, a member led organisation of people from all over the world living in Tyneside many of whom are refugees and people seeking asylum in the UK.

Dr Michael Kendrick has spent over five decades in the fields of disability and mental health internationally as a consultant, evaluator, trainer, writer, senior government leader, public speaker, activist and mentor. He has an enduring interest in values based leadership and the building of capacity to enable good lives for people who have experienced social devaluation and mistreatment. He is part of many ongoing networks interested in change and progress.

Les Billingham is Assistant Director of Adult Services & Community Development, Thurrock Council, England. He had a career in commerce before starting work in social care in 1995. Les has been a major driving force behind Thurrock's whole system transformation programmes which is predicated on delivering a strengths and placed based approach. Les has a double first class degree in Political Theory and Philosophy.

Tania Sitch is Partnership Director Adults Health and Social Care Thurrock Council, England. She has had a varied career in nursing, Inspection and regulation, and health and social care leadership and management. Her passion has always been about trying to improve the way we support people and undo years of focusing on crisis, dependency and bureaucracy. She was sold on Local Area Coordination from the first time she heard about it and is proud to be part of the Thurrock Journey since 2013.

Joe Micheli is Head of Commissioning (Early Intervention, Prevention & Community Development), City of York, England. With 30 years experience in citizen engagement, Joe established York's first Local Area Coordination programme in 2016. A key leader in the international Cities of Service network, he was previously Head of Stronger Communities at Barnsley Council.

Councillor Mark Child has held Cabinet Member responsibilities for Social Services and Prevention on Swansea Council since 2012 and is currently Lord Mayor of Swansea, Wales. He leads Swansea's membership of WHO Healthy Cities and is a member of Swansea Bay University Health Board. He has a keen interest in enabling and encouraging citizens to live healthy and active lives.

151

Neil Woodhead is currently the Local Area Coordination Team Manager at Derby City Council a post he has held for the last eight years. Since 2012 Neil has been responsible for the development, delivery, expansion and day to day management of Derby's Local Area Coordination team. Prior to joining Derby City Council Neil was employed as a Learning Disability Nurse working in the very state institutions he now seeks to dismantle.

Jennie Cox is Senior Local Area Coordinator in York, England. Her background relates mainly to mental health, homelessness and criminal justice, before becoming a Local Area Coordinator in 2017. She has a strong passion for social justice and inclusion, which she has brought to the Local Area Coordination Network. Jennie is particularly interested in system change led by citizen experience and often describes Local Area Coordinators as 'Social innovators, Expert generalists and Specialists in thinking outside the box'.

Ewa Neal has worked in various public sector coordination and management roles for the past 16 years and is currently a Local Communities Coordination Manager in a number of regions in Western Australia. She has a Bachelor of Science in Social Work and a Masters in Human Rights. She has taken an active role in shaping contemporary human services, putting into practice her passion about community development, social justice and personalised supports.

Kathryn Humpston is a Local Area Coordinator for the area of Boulton, Derby City. She has worked within Social Care for 38 years and proud to have been a Local Area Coordinator for six of those.

Catherine Viney is Disability Services Manager with Baptcare in Tasmania, Australia and had led that agency's development and implementation of Local Area Coordination across two states, She is driven by a desire to contribute to a more equitable Australian society. She has worked for much of her career with people with disability, beginning as teacher in the early bilingual bicultural programs for Deaf children.

Mary Flynn is a Local Area Coordinator with Leicestershire County Council in the UK. Mary is alongside a community called South Wigston that sits on the border of Leicester city but is in Leicestershire. In the past 3 years she has been part of new community initiatives such as the community garden and helps individuals take back control of their lives.

Anne Robinson is a Local Area Coordinator in Swansea. She loves seeing the positive changes individuals can make to their lives. When not working, Anne enjoy living a quiet life with her partner and youngest daughter, and takes great pleasure from spending time with her granddaughter.

Kim Harris has been a Local Area Coordinator for Derby City since 2018. She feels the job is a gift for the curious and an opportunity to be the best version of herself every day. Kim is a passionate reader who enjoys seeing how life shapes great stories through the power of listening and conversation.

Sian Roderick is a Senior Lecturer and Deputy Director of Postgraduate Research in the School of Management at Swansea University, Wales. She is a member of the iLab Research Centre and Chairs a weekly multidisciplinary research think tank – Scientia, which is primarily concerned with the formulation and creation of positive impacts for individuals, communities and regions. Sian has led several evaluation projects into life science skills, youth development initiatives and community cohesion initiatives such as Local Area Coordination in the South Wales region.

Dr Gareth Davies is an Associate Professor and Deputy Head of Department in Swansea University's School of Management, with research interests in innovation management and regional economic development. He has also worked on a broad range of industry and government funded policy and practice projects, across sectors from health & life sciences to construction.

Professor Jerry Tew worked as social worker before moving into academic teaching and research. He has undertaken research on recovery, personal budgets and 'whole family' approaches in mental health. He recently led a research programme for the Department of Health and Social Care on how Local Authorities were using strength-based and capacity building approaches to 'prevent, reduce or delay' the need for social care services.

Dr Sandhya Duggal is a research fellow based in the School of Social Policy, at the University of Birmingham. She has expertise in public health and adult social care, and is currently a co-investigator on a research project funded by the School for Social Care Research (NIHR), exploring the process and impact of implementing combinations of asset/strength-based approaches within adult social care.

Prof Joe Cook is Chair in Organizational Behaviour / Human Resource Management at the University of Hull. Her research interests include cross sectoral dialogue between public, private and third sectors alongside expertise in gender, migration and ageing. She is an experienced participatory action researcher utilising these methods since 2000. Her more recent projects focus upon social care, coproduction and community engagement. With current projects commissioned by the ESRC, NIHR and the Office for Civil Society.

Tania Loosley-Smith is a passionate public servant with over 25 years reform and leadership experience in housing and human services. A year into leading the Local Communities Coordination prototype in Western Australia, she describes it as the singly most powerful initiative she's ever seen in terms of positive, collective impacts for people, communities and government.

Dr WONG Sweet Fun is the Chief Transformation Officer and the Deputy Chairman, Medical Board (Population Health) at Yishun Health, National Healthcare Group in Singapore. A geriatrician actively involved for 20 years in preventive geriatrics, promotion of health, fitness and ageing-in-place for community-dwelling older adults, she leads population health improvement initiatives for the 550,000 residents living in the north of Singapore.

153

Evon CHUA is Senior Manager at the department of Population Health & Community Transformation (PHCT) in Yishun Health (Singapore) and is operational lead of Local Area Coordination in Yishun. Evon's work involves building active, healthy and inclusive communities sustainably by facilitating citizen participation in health creation, complemented with a good balance of support and services. She manages the department's regional teams.

Wan Ling WOO is Senior Manager at the department of Population Health & Community Transformation (PHCT) in Yishun Health (Singapore). She built her foundation in in-patient and out-patient operations within the Department of Geriatric Medicine, before moving on to manage population health with her current department at PHCT. Currently, her focus area is on developing staff capacity, and creating a culture that supports a strengths-based approach.

Emma Shears has been a Local Area Coordinator since 2017, working and walking alongside people in Swansea. Passionate for people to explore and achieve their vision of a good life and for communities to thrive. Alongside this role, I am a registered psychotherapeutic counsellor working in a local community setting and private practice.

Prof Donna Hall CBE was CEO of Wigan Council, where she developed *The Wigan Deal*. A passionate feminist, Donna ensured the Council has a zero gender pay gap. She is the Chair of New Local and Bolton NHS Foundation Trust, an Honorary Professor of Politics at the University of Manchester and an adviser to Birmingham City Council and NHS England.

Inclusive Neighbourhoods Ltd

Ralph Broad (Director) first worked in partnership with Local Area Coordination in Western Australia in the mid 1990s, initially as a member of a multi-disciplinary 'Individual and Family Support' team in local communities and subsequently as a manager of disability services in a non-government organisation in Western Australia. This was invaluable in the future development of, and commitment to, effective partnership working between Local Area Coordination and government and non-government services in new international sites.

Alongside Eddie Bartnik, Ralph contributed to some early developments of Local Area Coordination in the early 2000s, before leading the development of Local Area Coordination in England and Wales and establishing the Local Area Coordination Network. Ralph has subsequently supported the development of Local Area Coordination in Western Australia, Singapore and now the Isle of Man, as well as wider conversations, workshops and conferences alongside colleagues in New Zealand, NDIS partner organisations across Australia and IIDL conferences.

Contact Ralph Broad at Inclusive Neighbourhoods (based in England)

Email: ralph@inclusiveneighbourhoods.co.uk

154

Website: www.inclusiveneighbourhoods.co.uk

For International Local Area Coordination development and technical support (outside England and Wales) please contact Ralph Broad or Eddie Bartnik.

Tamar Consultancy Pty Ltd

Founded in 2000 by Eddie Bartnik as Principal Consultant, Tamar Consultancy continues to provide a wide range of international consultancy services. Eddie has been continuously involved in Local Area Coordination from its inception in the late 1980s right through to the present. Further to his early role as state-wide Director of Local Area Coordination in Western Australia, Eddie has been supporting local, and international developments throughout Australia and in New Zealand, Northern Ireland, Scotland, Ireland, England and various interested countries in Europe and North America.

In addition to Local Area Coordination, Tamar provides a unique range of tailored services across disability and mental health, including strategy and program development, mentoring and evaluation. Eddie has long and deep experience in human services reform and transformation and the values and principles of Local Area Coordination run deeply through all of his work.

Contact Eddie Bartnik at Tamar Consultancy Pty Ltd (based in Australia)

Email: ebartnik@iinet.net.au

155

Local Area Coordination Network

The Local Area Coordination Network (at Community Catalysts CIC) is the home of Local Area Coordination in England and Wales. Led by its Director, Nick Sinclair, it has dedicated resources to help bring sites together to reflect, learn and grow together. There are various sub-networks within the overall Network including a research network, leaders' network and Local Area Coordinator's reflective learning groups.

It is also the development agency for new sites (typically local authorities) wishing to implement Local Area Coordination in England and Wales. It supports new sites and their partners in all aspects of their design and development from initial concept inception right through to ongoing Network membership and support.

Contact Nick Sinclair at the Local Area Coordination Network (based in England)

Email: Nick.sinclair@communitycatalysts.co.uk

Website: www.lacnetwork.org

Centre for Welfare Reform

The Centre for Welfare Reform is an independent research and development network. Its aim is to transform the current welfare state so that it supports citizenship, family and community. It works by developing and sharing social innovations and influencing government and society to achieve necessary reforms.

To find out more go to www.centreforwelfarereform.org

To find out about Citizen Network and to join as an individual or a group visit: www.citizen-network.org

156

Relevant Publications

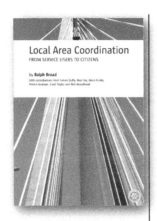

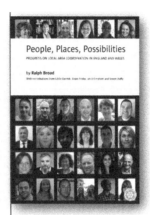

LOCAL AREA COORDINATION

Ralph Broad sets out the case for changing the whole approach of the social care system in England and Wales.

PEOPLE, PLACES, POSSIBILITIES

This report outlines the progress made in implementing Local Area Coordination in England and Wales between 2012 and 2015.

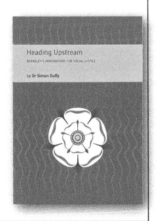

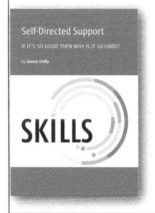

157

HEADING UPSTREAM

A report on how Barnsley Council have been increasing social justice by redistributing power and resources to local citizens, families and communities.

SELF-DIRECTED SUPPORT

The global movement towards self-directed support, or independent living, has been in progress for 50 years or more. So why has progress been so slow?

Lightning Source UK Ltd.
Milton Keynes UK
UKHW052158290821
389675UK00004B/66